"*A Polyvagal Informed Approach to Therapeutic Work with Children & Young People* by Karen O'Neill and Tara McDonald offers an insightful and compassionate guide for therapists, teachers, and parents seeking to understand and apply the Polyvagal framework in supporting the well-being of children and young individuals. Through compelling narratives told in the voices of children, readers witness the theory in action, enhancing understanding and relatability. With clear explanations, practical examples, and actionable strategies, this book delves into the nuanced interplay between the autonomic nervous system, social engagement, and emotional regulation. Through case studies and interventions rooted in play and metaphor, readers gain insights into navigating complex emotions, trauma, and developmental challenges. This essential resource emphasizes safety, co-regulation, and healthy nervous system development, offering hope and resilience in the face of adversity."

Stephen W. Porges, *PhD Distinguished University Scientist & Founding Director of Traumatic Stress Research Consortium, Kinsey Institute*

"This book is a really useful resource for a wide range of therapists and other professionals working with children. It explains Porges' theories and potential applications very well, but more than that, it provides a solid foundation for linking an understanding of the nervous system with other essential aspects of therapeutic work, such as transference and countertransference, metaphor, and play. The authors do this by using easy to understand clinical examples alongside solid helpful tools that practitioners will be grateful for."

Graham Music, *Consultant Child & Adolescent Psychotherapist, Tavistock Centre, Author, and Trainer*

"Karen and Tara's book, '*A Polyvagal Informed Approach to Therapeutic Work with Children & Young People*' is exceptional in simplifying the Polyvagal Theory. Their book brilliantly delves into how leveraging play as a therapeutic approach gets to the root of important concepts, fostering profound healing and deeper connections in therapy. It navigates complex ideas making them accessible and relevant to readers of all backgrounds. This book is a resource for anyone seeking knowledge and practical ways of implementing the Polyvagal Theory."

Jackie Flynn, *Licensed Psychotherapist, Registered Play Therapist, certified EMDR Therapist, EMDR Consultant*

W0113101

A Polyvagal Informed Approach to Therapeutic Work with Children and Young People

A Polyvagal Informed Approach to Therapeutic Work with Children and Young People presents a guide to best supporting children and young people through a polyvagal lens.

Through this neurophysiological framework of the Polyvagal Theory, the authors consider why children adopt protective strategies, unravelling the mysteries of the nervous system, emotions, and social connection. Linking aspects of attachment theory, developmental trauma, and adverse childhood experiences, the authors explore what shapes behaviour. They delve into perspectives of play and metaphor within the context of the Polyvagal Theory, utilising six storytellers who bring this theory to life, embodying real struggles and highlighting the adaptations children make for survival. Throughout this book, clear explanations, practical examples, and actionable strategies are offered to help the reader to understand and apply a polyvagal framework when working with children and young people.

This text is an accessible and important resource for all qualified child therapists, trainees, and professionals interested in the mental health of children and young people.

Karen O'Neill is an adult psychotherapist, child therapist, parent-infant therapist, and Eye Movement Desensitization and Reprocessing (EMDR) Europe Accredited Practitioner. Based in the UK, she offers psychotherapy to individuals as well as clinical supervision and consultancy work. Her specialist interest is parent-child dyads to strengthen the relationship between them.

Tara McDonald is a child therapist, adult psychotherapist, and clinical supervisor based in the UK. She works with individuals through a polyvagal and attachment-focused lens. Her passion is in supporting parents and carers who might be experiencing difficulties or hurt in their journey as a parent.

A Polyvagal Informed Approach to Therapeutic Work with Children and Young People

Karen O'Neill
Tara McDonald

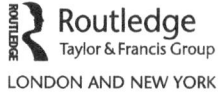
Routledge
Taylor & Francis Group

LONDON AND NEW YORK

Designed cover image: © Burcu Musselwhite

First published 2025
by Routledge
4 Park Square, Milton Park, Abingdon, Oxon OX14 4RN

and by Routledge
605 Third Avenue, New York, NY 10158

Routledge is an imprint of the Taylor & Francis Group, an informa business

© 2025 Karen O'Neill and Tara McDonald

British Library Cataloguing-in-Publication Data
A catalogue record for this book is available from the British Library

ISBN: 9781032535524 (hbk)
ISBN: 9781032535517 (pbk)
ISBN: 9781003412571 (ebk)

DOI: 10.4324/9781003412571

Typeset in Times New Roman
by KnowledgeWorks Global Ltd.

Contents

Foreword

It is an exciting time to be a part of the field of play therapy. We understand so much more about what is happening inside our child clients as well as what is happening inside of ourselves as we are facilitating play and healing.

As a play therapist, supervisor, creator of Synergetic Play Therapy, and play therapy trainer for over 20 years, it has been truly inspiring to watch the play therapy field adapt and shift as new insights about the brain, the nervous system, and ultimately children's behaviour have emerged.

With each new understanding, we are asked to pause and to question what we think we know and to become curious about what parts of our thinking, interventions, and ultimately paradigm need to shift. This questioning is not easy, as it bumps up against what we think we understand and where we might feel competent. Integration of new ideas and insights such as Stephen Porges' Polyvagal Theory, the focus of this book, requires us to go back to the beginning and reassemble a new way of thinking about play and how healing occurs.

As often happens with new ideas and theories, the translation into practical application can at times be challenging. In this book, Karen O'Neill and Tara McDonald have risen to the task and have taken this significant theory and demonstrated exactly how to weave it into the playroom. With compassion, tenderness, and a deep care of the reader, they offer a way for play therapists to think about Polyvagal Theory in the playroom.

Karen and Tara are committed to the advancement of the play therapy field and even more inspiring, committed to the growth and development of play therapists. In this book, they bring to life Polyvagal Theory as we follow the journeys of six children, Amira, Teddy, Tom, Hannah, Emma, and Ezra. We learn to think about their situations from a polyvagal lens and ultimately how to help.

One of the most interesting aspects of this book is the comprehensive approach taken to help play therapists hold a larger framework of what might be happening for the child. From discussions on the autonomic nervous system, adverse childhood experiences, developmental trauma, attachment ruptures, and COVID, no stone is left unturned. As further support, Karen and Tara present various handouts and visuals. These are extremely useful tools for treatment conceptualisation, supporting caregivers and understanding what is happening inside of ourselves.

I would like to emphasise the importance of embodying what we learn in this book. It is one thing to learn how to apply a theory into the playroom, but it is another thing entirely to try the theory on in order to feel the theory. To take a theory such as the Polyvagal Theory and see how it comes to life inside of our own bodies offers us a unique understanding and perspective. As such, my invitation is to continuously turn inward as you read this book. Read the information, do the exercises that are offered, and reflect on how this theory plays out in your own body and in your relationships.

One of the most important understandings that has emerged in the play therapy field is the recognition that we are deeply impacted by a child's play, stories, and behaviours. Polyvagal Theory and the information in this book not only offer us a window into how we can help our child clients but also build resiliency within ourselves in the midst of our own activation.

The reality is that when we are in play therapy sessions, we feel. Much of this can be attributed to the mirror neuron system, as this system is set up to help us feel what other people feel. The significance of this for all play therapists is that when a child is playing and telling stories, we pick up on the child's nonverbal and verbal cues, which is directly linked to what is happening inside of their nervous system. As we pick up on these cues, somatic shifts simultaneously occur within us giving us information about what might be going on for the child.

As amazing as this process is, it also means that play therapists will feel the activation whether they want to or not. As a result, play therapists are in a very vulnerable position. This is where understanding and applying Polyvagal Theory and the information in this book becomes paramount. Without our ability to understand our own activation and access our ventral state, we put ourselves at risk of internalising the activation and emotional experiences we are experiencing setting us up for vicarious trauma and compassion fatigue.

As mentioned, it is an extraordinary time to be a play therapist as new information is emerging guiding us towards deeper understandings of the healing process, for our child clients and also within ourselves. Polyvagal Theory and information on the brain is reminding us of the importance of being with the child rather than doing something to the child. It is highlighting the need to get curious and to question what we think we already know. In many ways, the information in this book is a call to action to see our clients from a new lens. It is an invitation to go underneath labels, stories, and behaviours and to become curious about the wisdom that exists inside each client and in our own patterns of activation. It is time to relook at what we think we know about what is happening inside of ourselves and our clients.

Lisa Dion, LPC, RPT-S, Creator of Synergetic Play Therapy

Acknowledgements

Together, we thank all of those who have guided and mentored us over many years. We celebrate the very talented Burcu Musselwhite who has illustrated this book.

Our appreciation is extended to Lisa Dion for her ongoing support. Graham Music and Jackie Flynn, thank you for endorsing our work. Finally, we send our gratitude to Dr Stephen Porges for taking the time to offer feedback and guidance which we feel have enhanced *A Polyvagal Informed Approach to Therapeutic Work with Children and Young People*.

Karen O'Neill

I am grateful to all the wise people that I have known in my life. Every one of you have contributed to the landscape of my nervous system and the 'novelty' of this book. Tara, you have my upmost respect.

Professionally, I offer my appreciation to clients and professionals whom I have worked with. Moments of richness and meaning into your worlds have shown me another way.

Personally, I express my love and gratitude to my rainbow family who bring their own colour and vibrancy to relationships. Finally, to my beloved grandparents whose gifts I treasure within my heart and my darling husband who has continued to wait patiently in the wings to catch me with care, kindness, and love.

Tara McDonald

It never occurred to me that I might one day sit and write a book, and I would never have considered doing this alone. Thank you Karen for your creativity, partnership, friendship, and many opportunities for personal growth.

This book is a culmination of the years I have spent learning from my greatest teachers, the children and families who have entrusted me with their stories. I have learned so much from you and have nothing but gratitude for your tenacity, bravery, and mission to find playfulness again. Your courage and commitment inspire me every day.

My work has been moulded, formed, and influenced by so many brilliant hearts and minds. I am moved to thank two women in particular who demonstrate mastery in the field of children's mental health. Elaine McCullogh, I learn so much from you; our walks in the park have sustained me throughout this process. Steph Lethlean, even though we are on the opposite sides of the globe, you remain a huge inspiration and walk the walk, regulating and coregulating as you go.

Throughout my life, I have had two consistent cheerleaders who understand friendship and connection like no other. I have endless gratitude for Susannah Phillips and the lifelong sisterhood a tin of Quality Street gave us at the tender age of 11. Carole Crumplin, it all started on a hay bale, and I have loved and laughed ever since.

To my incredible family. A big, dispersed brood who navigate relationships in unique ways; thank you all for your belief and support. And finally, to the most important humans in my world, total appreciation for the amazing Tim, my bedrock, and our two brilliant and kind children Alfie and Flo. I couldn't have done this without you.

Introduction

We met in 2013 and connected at a Family Therapy training and have always felt very aligned personally and professionally. We have had a similar journey as psychotherapists and counselling practitioners, both originally qualifying to work with adults before moving into child, adolescent, and family work. Our qualifications, knowledge base, and skills are varied to work therapeutically with different age range clients, which is underpinned with reflective practice. Our understanding of theory to work safely is informed by our work as Adult Psychotherapists, Child Therapists, Dyadic Family Therapists, and Trauma Informed Therapists.

We became aware of the Polyvagal Theory soon after meeting and had many discussions about how Stephen Porges' concepts offered an additional lens to think about how our clients experienced the world. Taking the earliest opportunity to access training with both Stephen Porges and Deb Dana, we became motivated to learning as much as we could about the Polyvagal Theory, the Vagus Nerve, and Autonomic Nervous System.

There are very few books written to help and guide child therapists in their clinical work and become Polyvagal informed. Inspired, we decided to write our first book together *A Polyvagal Informed Approach to Therapeutic Work with Children and Young People* for those working therapeutically with children and young people. We hope that professionals and therapists from all disciplines will find our book informative and stimulating, encouraging rich discussion about Porges theory.

At its core, *A Polyvagal Informed Approach to Therapeutic Work with Children and Young People* is an invitation to explore the depths of the human experience through the lens of the Polyvagal Theory. As therapists, educators, and advocates of child mental health, we have witnessed first-hand the challenges that children and young people face which vary greatly, depending on their individual circumstances, family dynamics, experiences, and needs.

An invitation is offered to readers to embrace curiosity, openness, and a spirit of exploration. We provide a tapestry of ideas that link the complex interplay between our physiological state and our psychological well-being. Our ideas and insights are presented as we introduce you to four new concepts that we have developed: *ANS 'A' States, The Needs Paradox®, Symbolic Repair©, and The Super Protector©*.

DOI. 10.4324/9781003412571-1

In addition, we present two new assessment tools designed to facilitate goal setting and inform the planning of therapy and therapeutic interventions: *Child Social Engagement Capacity Questionnaire© (CSECQ)* and *Physiological Markers Checklist© (PMC)*. These concepts and assessment tools will be discussed in the most relevant chapters to enhance further depth of understanding and application to clinical work. They are available to download for free at: https://www.pipsolutions.co.uk.

Throughout this book, clear explanations, practical examples, and actionable strategies are offered to help the reader to understand and apply a polyvagal framework when working with children and young people.

We hope that *A Polyvagal Informed Approach to Therapeutic Work with Children and Young People* stimulates your interest as you contemplate thought-provoking questions about yourself and others. As you embark on this journey of discovery with us, together we will unravel the mysteries of the nervous system, emotions, and social connection.

Chapter 1

Introducing the Polyvagal Theory

The Polyvagal Theory is the science of safety. As humans, we are on a persistent quest for safety and have evolved to rely on trusted connections with others. Therapists working with children and young people are only too aware of the impact an unsafe world has on their well-being. Our efforts are concentrated on returning stability to our clients. We seek ways in which they can process what has happened to them. We share unifying goals to leave those we support with an experience of nurture; to have an integrated self, able to trust in relationships and live their lives with playful curiosity. The Polyvagal Theory serves therapists by offering a framework within which we can truly appreciate our clients and their journey. Their behaviours, however incongruous, demonstrate a tenacious desire to manage past experiences, protect themselves, and survive. "Safety is the treatment" (Badenoch, 2018a).

The first writings about heart rate rhythm and the concept of heart rate variability (HRV) can be traced back to the ancient Greek physician and scientist Herophilius (ca. 335–280 BC). During the early 1960s, psychophysiology was emerging as an interdisciplinary science. At the crossroads of several disciplines, psychophysiology is a branch of psychology that focuses on processes of thoughts, emotions, and behaviours influenced by physiological responses of the nervous, endocrine, cardiovascular, and respiratory systems.

In 1966, Stephen Porges was studying for a master's degree at graduate school and became interested in the electrical activity of the heart and measuring heart rate. Porges and his mentor, David Raskin, published a paper 'Respiratory and heart rate components of attention' (1969) that quantified HRV and breathing patterns. At the intersection of psychology, neuroscience, and evolutionary biology, Porges developed a range of tools to monitor autonomic state whilst continuing to research the link between HRV and respiratory sinus arrhythmia (RSA) as markers of parasympathetic regulation. His research into preterm newborns demonstrated the dynamic interplay between the sympathetic and parasympathetic branches of the autonomic nervous system (ANS). The presence of a depressed RSA showed the immaturity of the infant's ventral vagal pathway, impacting the capacity of the ventral vagal complex to regulate HRV effectively. Pointing to infant vulnerabilities in managing stress and environmental challenges, both are exacerbated in the

DOI: 10.4324/9781003412571-2

neonatal intensive care unit (NICU). Furthermore, feeding babies show that the 'suck-swallow-breathe-vocalize behaviours' involve the ventral vagal complex, nervous system efficiency, and effective coordination encompassing "vagal regulation of the heart through the ventral vagal pathways" (Porges, 2021).

Simply put, during inhalation, the heart rate typically increases whilst during exhalation the heart rate decreases. RSA measures cardiac vagal tone and its connections to emotional regulation, stress responses, and social engagement. It is considered as an index of parasympathetic nervous system activity and the influence of the vagus nerve on heart modulation. Vagal tone and RSA are closely related, as they both reflect the functioning of the vagus nerve in regulating the heart rate.

In 1994, Dr Stephen Porges introduced the scientific community to his Polyvagal Theory during his presidential address to the Society for Psychophysiological Research in Atlanta, Georgia. This was the culmination of approximately 30 years of research in identifying heart rate patterns as a way of offering insights into autonomic function and overall health. He proposed that the ANS is a state response with two branches of the vagus nerve, with each supporting different "adaptive behavioural strategies" (Porges, 2007). HRV serves as a non-invasive marker relating to mental and physical health-related processes.

Alongside Stephen Porges, Deb Dana is a founder of Polyvagal Institute. Together, they have co-authored *Clinical Applications of the Polyvagal Theory: The Emergence of Polyvagal-Informed Therapies* (2018). Dana is a licenced clinical social worker and psychotherapist. Her work emerged from 2015 onwards, and she is credited with bringing the Polyvagal Theory to the attention of counsellors, therapists, and health professionals. An author in her own right, Dana has published several books whereby she has taken the principles of Polyvagal Theory and translated them into a language that can be understood and applied by clinicians.

In 2018, she published her first book, *Polyvagal Theory in Therapy*, which helped curious professionals understand and integrate the theory's principles into their clinical work. Dana offered a neurophysiological framework to understand automatic and adaptive actions, emphasising the importance of understanding the nervous system's role in shaping emotional and behavioural responses. Offering practitioners a way of familiarising themselves with their nervous systems, her seminal work has generalised the concepts of the Polyvagal Theory within the field of Adult Psychotherapy. Her influence can be seen throughout this book as concepts are extended and built up for use with children and young people and their families. Adopting a polyvagal framework insists that the therapist is as curious about their own internal experience, as that of their clients.

Contemporary psychotherapy has been significantly influenced by theories and frameworks focused on neuroscience, particularly in the last three decades. Currently, it seems we are undergoing a small-scale revolution regarding the intricate link between the brain and body. The progression of therapeutic approaches has shifted our emphasis from behaviour-centric perspectives to a heightened focus on affect. By incorporating insights from neuroscience, biology, and physics, our comprehension has moved beyond the simplistic notion of 'I think, therefore, I behave', urging us to entertain the idea of 'I feel, therefore, I behave, and then perhaps I think, if possible!'

A polyvagal framework lends itself to all therapeutic modalities, whether you offer creative therapy or talking therapy. This model helps us understand that it is how we are, not how we work that will have a greater impact on client outcomes. It is through signalling repeated cues of safety that clients' defensive systems are dampened and social behaviour is facilitated. It is through co-regulation and reciprocity that clients will experience a sense of connectedness. It is through attunement that clients will feel understood. It is through our capacity to modulate their window of tolerance that clients will gain awareness of their own internal states. The offering of these conditions has the potential to intentionally influence our clients' nervous systems, reorganising their neural expectation of threat to one of safety.

Maslow identified that safety is a basic need, second only to the necessary physiological requirements for human survival, and a precursor to our innate drive for love, esteem, and self-actualisation. The therapeutic world is aptly preoccupied with discussions around how we can help clients feel safe and how we might create safe spaces. Ultimately, we are concerning ourselves with how we can support our clients to have an internal and subjective felt sense that they are protected from harm or danger.

The term 'felt sense' was coined by philosopher and psychotherapist Eugene Gendlin. He explained that a felt sense is a bodily experience:

A felt sense is not a mental experience but a physical one. A bodily awareness of a situation or person or event. An internal aura that encompasses everything you feel and know about a given subject at a given time, encompasses it and communicates it to you all at once, rather than detail by detail.

(Gendlin, 1978)

The Polyvagal Theory develops this understanding through a neurophysiological lens. Porges (2017, 2023) emphasises that there are two important concepts related to feeling safe that we, as therapists, must hold: the absence of threat does not make a person feel safe. Feeling safe is dependent on the ANS remaining out of a system of defence, so it can detect cues of safety via the process of neuroception.

Crucially, a person's felt sense of safety equates to their perception of whether someone or something is safe, regardless of the facts. It is about how the body feels. It is not automatic and does not appear when presented with a situation or person that means no harm. We cannot presume to know what is biologically safe for our clients, and the significance of our ability to self-regulate and remain truly authentic throughout the process cannot be overstated. Soma *et al.* (2020) suggest that "psychotherapy is a particular form of a close, emotion laden interpersonal relationship with the explicit goal of one individual influencing the psychological well-being of another". This positive influence will only happen through right brain to right brain non-verbal communication.

Our right brain is relational. It develops functionality earlier than the left, co-inciding with the developmental timetable of attachment. As such, it is the keeper of our implicit memories. Strongly connected to the ANS (Schore, 2009), our client's right brain is looking at how we behave, respond, and regulate ourselves.

Applying the Polyvagal Theory to child therapy requires the therapist to be observant of their own internal experience, whilst supporting the needs of their client as "there can be no openness to the child's experience if there is no openness to one's own experience" (Tucci *et al.*, 2018). If we are alert to the shifting sensations in our own bodies, we gain insight into what the client is feeling. Due to children's right brain bias, they will typically be communicating their experience through shared bodily sensations rather than language. The Polyvagal Theory develops on the concept of somatic transference, which refers to the involuntary conveyance of emotions, memories, and physical sensations from one individual to another. Within this interaction, the inner experiences of our clients manifest in ourselves. An awareness of our own triggers helps us consider, 'is this my stuff, or theirs?' If we recognise what our own body needs to return to a regulated and socially engaged position, we can apply this in the moment within the therapy session, modelling and mirroring the pathway back to regulation.

Holding in mind the biological explanation as to why our clients demonstrate positive and negative reactions whilst interacting with others and their environment removes the demand for hurt children and young people to rationalise why they behave the way they do. Feeling safe is a biological process that is supported by regulating relationships.

The offering of a therapeutic relationship will be a novelty to most of the children and young people we work with. It is our understanding that Porges' description of novelty relates to safety and security; he explains, "those who are bold and seek novelty may also be those who have or who have had the most efficient pathways back to safety" (2017).

In almost all cases, children and young people are referred to therapy due to their inability to self-regulate. From a polyvagal lens, self-regulation can be understood as the capacity for the nervous system to maintain a feeling of safety "in the absence of receiving cues of safety from another person" (Porges, 2017). A polyvagal framework helps us consider whether the child has the capacity to return 'home' to a regulated position, following a felt sense of threat. We are designed to respond and react hierarchically, according to the perception of threat when something upsets or frightens us. Those autonomic reactions keep us safe. A strong vagal tone returns us to a regulated position once the danger is past. Regardless of their presenting issue, whether it is grief, friendship issues, difficulties with sleep, inattention, or separation anxiety, a contributing factor in a referral being made to you is that the child is unable to return to a state of homeostasis. Their nervous system is stuck in a state of hyper- or hypo-arousal.

We offer our concept of ANS 'A' States in relation to hierarchy as a quick and understandable guide to how the ANS responds to neuroception of safety or danger through three pathways of response: ventral, sympathetic, and dorsal. These responses work in a specified order and can only be moved through the hierarchy ladder in sequence.

Some of the children and young people we work with have lived through abuse or neglect in their early childhood, resulting in developmental trauma. A child's capacity to socially engage is determined by their lived experience and neural expectation developed during significant windows of opportunity. Children and young people whose nervous systems have developed in a threatening environment will adapt and change in order to survive. Their ANS will be altered to defend themselves in service of protection. They will not look for connection as a solution to their distress. Rather, they will utilise historical responses that have led to their survival, be that running away, fighting, screaming, or shutting down. In the past, the response matched the threat. As an example, we might think about a baby who learnt not to cry because their mother became overwhelmed and left them in another room until they stopped seeking nurture and shut down. Fast-forward 5 years, and that same child now lives with their grandmother, who tries her best to demonstrate love and compassion. Yet, this little girl remains persistently withdrawn, resisting attempts at connection. In the context of the here and now, the threat has been removed, but the child's autonomic response to the offer of comfort and closeness remains 'as if' it is a threat.

The Needs Paradox® is a framework to consider the psychobiological conflict children and young people who have lived through developmental trauma may encounter when they are offered therapeutic care, attunement, and co-regulation. The therapist's role is to interactively repair original wounds through implicit affect regulation whilst working alongside the child's protective adaptations that were necessitated in service of survival.

In order to survive, strategies have been developed to negotiate life and rely on a fractured self. Adult attention has historically been dangerous, harmful, and unreliable. Therapeutic intervention through a polyvagal lens honours and respects the strategies a child has taken. Porges (2022) suggests that "Polyvagal Theory proposes that social connectedness is tantamount to stating that our body feels safe in proximity with another". These children and young people will need us to give them repeated cues of safety. Our voices, facial expressions, breath, and body movements communicate whether we are safe or threatening.

Just as the brain is continually changing in response to experiences and the environment, our ANS is likewise engaged and can be intentionally influenced (Dana, 2018).

As a relatively new theory, direct evidence of its applicability to human behaviour and physiology continues to be documented. There are criticisms of the Polyvagal Theory. These criticisms tend to focus on points unrelated to the principles of the theory (Porges, 2023) such as concerns that the theory oversimplifies the complex interactions within the ANS and questions around whether the vagus nerve is a primary mediator of social behaviour and emotional regulation. However, these challenges are not consistent with the theory's propositions and come without a competing hypothesis, which would have enabled further scientific scrutiny. Validated by current neuroscience and cited in several thousand peer-reviewed publications, the Polyvagal Theory is best upheld by its relatability to the human experience. We maintain that the theory remains an invaluable and practical framework for therapists. Its innovative perspective on the ANS and its influence on emotional and social behaviour provides therapists with powerful tools for understanding and working with children and young people.

Neurophysiology cannot be ignored. Modern neuroscientists, psychologists, and attachment theorists take an interdisciplinary perspective when considering mental and emotional health. As noted by Antonio Damasio, "we are not thinking machines that feel; rather, we are feeling machines that think" (1994). The Polyvagal Theory offers a new lens to consider ANS dynamics in the context of emotional regulation and social engagement.

Within the chapters that follow, we will provide a tapestry of ideas that link the complex interplay between our physiological state and our psychological well-being. We commence by providing a clear understanding of the Polyvagal Theory and how the ANS emphasises the role of the vagus nerve and acts as an internal surveillance system, operating on a pre-thought basis, shaping our experience of safety and our ability to connect with others. As we journey through the foundational concepts of the Polyvagal Theory, we explore the three distinct branches of the ANS: the ventral vagal complex, the sympathetic nervous system, and the dorsal vagal complex. You will learn how these pathways influence our responses to threat, safety, and social connection, shaping our emotional experiences and interpersonal relationships.

Autonomic states and levels of defence have a physiological presentation. An awareness of these indicators of autonomic states, such as facial expressions, breath, pupil dilation, and tone of voice, can assist you in evaluating a client's openness or resistance to connection. To help you consider how your clients present, we introduce the Physiological Markers Checklist© (PMC), which can be a useful addition in case conceptualisation, goal setting, and planning the next steps in therapy.

We introduce our six storytellers, Amira, Teddy, Tom, Hannah, Emma, and Ezra, to help bring the theory alive. Throughout the book, their experiences will facilitate your understanding of key concepts and how to apply the theory to your work. They are not real cases but a union of the many children and young people we have worked with over the years. Through their stories, this book offers you an additional way of thinking about how you work and what the children you support need from you. We consider the various ways behaviours seen in our clients are manifested and shaped. Discussing adverse childhood experiences (ACEs), attachment, and developmental trauma through a polyvagal lens, we emphasise their profound impact on ANS development.

Neuroception of safety and co-regulation will be discussed through the lens of play as a neural exercise. As a vehicle of expression, play and metaphorical processes support the ANS without fear, triggering protective responses and thus supporting physiological states. We help you apply an understanding of the framework of the Polyvagal Theory and therapeutic work at different stages of the therapeutic process.

Interpersonal dynamics of transference and countertransference in the therapeutic relationship are contemplated, recognising these processes as integral to the therapeutic dyad. This is particularly relevant in the context of the COVID-19 pandemic, where therapists had to adjust to the changing landscape as the autonomic needs for safety were challenged due to extended periods of lockdown and social isolation.

You are invited to think about how therapists must become familiar with their autonomic states to effectively engage with clients whilst maintaining personal well-being. We consider how therapist burnout often stems from neglecting the regulation of their own nervous systems. Parents, caregivers, and teachers are not forgotten. We discuss how adults can be helped to better understand and respond to the neurobiological underpinnings of stress and engagement in the home and the classroom.

Symbolic Repair© is offered to consider the notion that within an attuned therapeutic relationship, the therapist can stimulate the experience of nurture in infancy. Constructed through a relational system using metaphor and imaginative play 'symbolic repair' is defined as: "the application of attachment principles to psychotherapeutic processes through metaphor and imaginative play, whereby the child client can internalise a new model of good enough parent through the dynamic processes of the therapeutic dyad" (O'Neill, 2023).

As child therapists, we may ask parents to partake in parent–child sessions, or it may be mandated. If the parent is emotionally unavailable or unwilling to engage in a therapist–parent alliance, change for the child may be limited, and the parent–child relationship may be compromised. In the context of the Polyvagal Theory, when parent–child therapy is not possible, symbolic repair© can offer a "sensitive, playful, therapeutic relationship", whereby "there is the opportunity for a child to rewrite a previously painful experience in a new way" (Daniel & Trevarthen, 2017, p. 148). By fostering safety, connection, and regulation through metaphor and imaginative play, the therapist can help rewire the child or young person's nervous system, which can be experienced through a new model of therapy called 'symbolic repair' (O'Neill, 2023).

We also think about first meetings, offering additions to a typical intake process. You are introduced to the Child Social Engagement Capacity Questionnaire© (CSECQ), a tool designed to support therapists to begin the process of formulating an understanding of their client's autonomic responses to the environment. This assists you with case conceptualisation in the context of three important concepts: (1) goal setting, (2) adult mentalisation, and (3) psychoeducational needs.

Throughout the book, we offer a variety of activities and exercises to help explore your ANS. We encourage curiosity about your individual experiences of each state and provide tools to navigate stress-induced responses. We have set ourselves the goal to guide you to return to connection in the face of dysregulation and integrate this self-awareness into your therapy sessions.

By acknowledging that behaviours and reactions are automatic and shaped by the nervous system's reaction to perceived threats, empathy and understanding can naturally develop. Sharing this knowledge with our clients has the capacity to reduce self-blame and grow self-understanding. To support professionals to explain the Polyvagal Theory to their clients, we have created The Super Protector©. This simple illustrated guide provides professionals with clear, step-by-step instructions, utilising creative activities and strategies to help clients become familiar with how their systems work and how to read bodily signals when moving into protective responses.

As we move to the final chapter, we summarise our thoughts in the hope that we have illuminated the Polyvagal Theory in a way that offers a deeper understanding of what it means to be human and the need for ANS safety. Being Polyvagal-informed affords a framework whereby therapists can conceptualise and consider techniques or strategies to support children, young people, parents, and professionals. For the remainder of this book, we will use the terms 'child' or 'children' to describe a person under the age of 18 and 'parent(s)' to describe an adult responsible for the child.

Chapter 2

Our Six Storytellers

To bring the Polyvagal Theory to life, we have recruited the help of Amira, Teddy, Tom, Hannah, Emma, and Ezra. Our Six Storytellers aren't real individuals. They are based on the different children, young people, and families that we have had the privilege to work with. Ranging in age, ethnicity, family constellation, and life experience, they have all adapted to survive their unique set of circumstances.

Some of these children have been labelled or dismissed as unmanageable. They tell a story of survival and should be honoured. Their bodies are vessels of a knowing stuckness and if we listen closely, all the information is there. They are warriors.

Hurt children must never be met with judgement. Looking through a polyvagal lens, we understand that their behaviours have been borne out of necessity. Our Six Storytellers demonstrate how the autonomic nervous system operates in service of survival. By delving into these cases, you have the opportunity to witness the theory in action, making it more relatable and accessible. These examples not only enhance understanding but also enable a more nuanced exploration of the intricate interplay between the autonomic nervous system, social engagement, and emotional regulation.

These portrayals aim to capture the diverse challenges and dynamics encountered within professional practice. Their stories help us to share ways of working through a polyvagal lens, giving you an illustration of the broader themes and patterns observed in the clinical space.

DOI: 10.4324/9781003412571-3

Amira

Age:	1 Years old

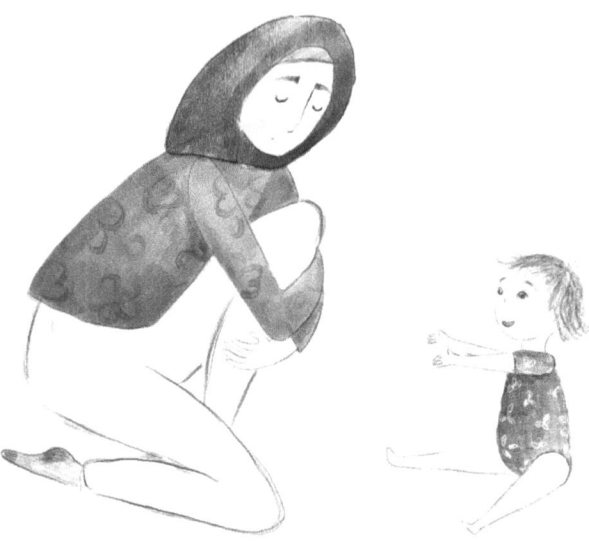

Figure 2.1 Amira.

Family Dynamics

Amira lives with her mum and dad, Layla, and Ali. They are both in their late thirties, they met 6 months before becoming pregnant with Amira. This was Layla's first pregnancy; Ali has an older daughter who is aged 8 years from a previous relationship. He does not see his daughter; it is known that there was domestic violence from Ali towards his ex-partner.

Layla's Mum and older brother do not live locally. Layla has not seen either since meeting Ali. She was very close to her dad who died 3 years ago. Ali had not been in contact with his adoptive parents since leaving home when he was 16 years old.

Developmental Milestones

It has been observed that Amira is a quiet baby, there are concerns about how she is vocally engaging. She does not laugh or babble. She does not vocalise any sounds and is not saying any words. Amira is of low weight for her age.

Additional Needs

Amira has not been diagnosed with any additional needs but there are concerns as to how she presents.

Medical History

Amira had severe reflux and colic for the first 6 months of her life. The GP prescribed medication but this led to constipation which she was treated for.

COVID-19 Experience

Amira was born during the first lockdown of COVID-19. Layla had an emergency caesarean section and described a traumatic birth. She did not have skin-to-skin contact with Amira after she was born as there were complications. Amira was quickly transferred to the Neonatal Infant Care Unit after birth (NICU).

Layla and Ali have no family or friend support networks. They live in a village and during COVID-19, they were isolated. All health appointments were online and there were no parent-baby groups due to the lockdowns. Although there is limited availability, face-to-face parent-infant groups have recommenced and are being offered within the locality. Layla does not want to attend any groups as she feels highly anxious, preferring to stay at home isolating herself from family members and others. Amira is on a Child in Need Plan because of concerns that her needs are not being met by Layla and Ali.

Reason for Referral

Amira has been referred to a local service that supports parents with their relationship with their infants. The referral was made by a professional involved with the family as they are concerned about Layla's bonding/connection with Amira. Layla has no concerns about her relationship with Amira and doesn't understand the purpose of the referral but agreed to it being made. Ali is worried about Amira and Layla's bonding. He believes that this was because of a lack of skin-to-skin contact between them when she was first born as, well as Amira's stay in NICU for the first 10 days of her life.

There are concerns that Amira is compliant and not able to express her needs. It has been observed that she uses her body to show her distress. She can present in any of the following ways: 'smiley', minimal eye contact with her parents, floppy, arching her body, engaging intensely with strangers.

Background Information

Layla and Ali live in a one-bedroom flat. They rely on benefits and often struggle to pay utility bills or afford to buy food. Layla has suffered from depression since adolescence and Ali was diagnosed with bipolar disorder in his late twenties. Both take medication and are under the care of mental health services.

Professionals are involved with the family. Regular meetings are held due to ongoing concerns about Layla's and Ali's parenting skills and capabilities. Amira has been described as a 'smiley baby' who rarely cries. Layla and Ali have been observed to respond to Amira differently. Layla has little engagement with Amira, rarely speaks or holds her. Whereas Ali is intrusive, has little awareness of personal boundaries and speaks loudly.

Case Conceptualisation

Professionals are concerned that Amira is not meeting her developmental milestones and that her needs are not being met. They have observed that Layla and Ali handle Amira very roughly, are not attentive, responsive, or sensitive to her needs.

Amira is an infant who communicates her distress through her body. In the presence of both parents, Amira can be 'smiley' and lack affect often presenting as compliant. With Layla, Amira smiles and tries to catch her mum's 'eye'. Amira is more animated with Layla and often moves her body and has more dribble in her mouth. When Layla notices this, she puts a muslin cloth in Amira's mouth to wipe it. Amira does not protest when Layla does this.

With Ali, Amira either arches her back or goes floppy. This is dependent on how Ali uses his body and the loudness of his voice. When Ali is intrusive or picking Amira up in a rough manner, she turns her head and avoids eye contact. Amira does not attempt to engage with Ali.

In terms of vagal tone, this appears to be underdeveloped as there are minimal opportunities provided by Layla or Ali to support Amira with this. With reference to hierarchy, we see that Amira tries to move into social engagement with Layla, but this is not reciprocated and often unsuccessful. Therefore, Amira often moves into sympathetic. With Ali, we see that Amira moves between sympathetic and dorsal. With both parents, Amira is under stress and her sense of neuroception leans towards cues of danger rather than cues of safety. Layla and Ali need input to support their parenting. Parent-infant observations and interventions are required to help Layla and Ali in their connection, bonding, and parenting of Amira.

Teddy

Age:	4 Years old

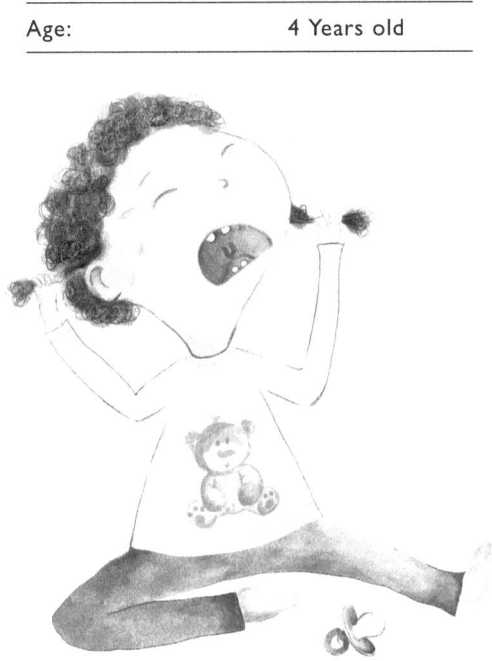

Figure 2.2 Teddy.

Family Dynamics

Teddy is an only child and has lived at home with his maternal grandparents since he was aged 18 months. Betty and Charles are in their early sixties and Teddy is the child of their daughter, Jemma. Betty is Teddy's full-time caregiver, Charles works in a factory.

Teddy was placed under a Special Guardianship Order (SGO) due to neglect as Jemma has continued to maintain a relationship with her partner who has convictions for drug dealing. Whilst with her current partner, Jemma has experienced severe domestic violence including rape. Social Services are involved with the family and the Police have been called on numerous occasions. Jemma feels unable to make a statement against her partner.

Developmental Milestones

Teddy was described by Health Visitors as having a flat head and unable to sit up unaided until he was 12 months old. It was documented that he appeared to be disconnected at times from his surroundings and environment. Since living with Betty and Charles, Teddy has reached his developmental milestones but is described as small for his aged.

Additional Needs

No additional needs have been identified for Teddy. Nursery staff reports that he is often distressed when his grandma leaves him at nursery and that it is difficult for them to calm him down. They describe how he flops onto the floor and cries like a baby. Betty is often called to collect Teddy from the nursery. As soon as she arrives it is noticeable that his distress levels reduce and that he calms down in her presence. Charles has stated that Teddy can have meltdowns at home, especially when his Mum visits.

Medical History

Teddy experienced neglect from his mum, Jemma which was one of the main reasons that he was placed in the care of Betty and Charles. He has a dummy and there are concerns that it is doing damage to his teeth. It has been noted that his top and bottom front teeth do not touch.

COVID-19 Experience

Betty and Charles found lockdown difficult as they were in a high-risk group and had to isolate. They saw very few people. Professionals remained in contact, all appointments were online.

Teddy did not see Jemma during the lockdown period. Teddy was offered a place at nursery but because Betty and Charles were shielding, he did not attend. They reported that Teddy was much more settled at home and had less meltdowns. For this reason, Betty and Charles felt that lockdown was a good thing.

Since the nursery has reopened, Teddy has struggled to settle. Betty has stated that there are more problems than there were before the lockdowns and social distancing. She is finding it difficult to get Teddy into nursery. There are days where Teddy is so distressed, and his meltdowns are so big that Betty takes him back home as she cannot cope with his behaviours in these moments.

Reason for Referral

Teddy was referred to Play Therapy because of his emotional distress and behaviours.

Everyone recognised that Teddy's early life experiences have impacted him. There are concerns that when he goes to school next year, his behaviours will not be managed. Currently, nobody knows what help or strategies Teddy needs, or even if they are available. There is worry that as he gets older, his behaviours will escalate.

Background Information

Jemma is aged 22 years; she is the youngest sibling. She has two older siblings, a brother who is 28 years old and a sister who is 32 years old.

Jemma became pregnant after a 'one-night stand' when she was 18 years old. She felt no connection to Teddy throughout her pregnancy and had gender disappointment.

Furthermore, she did not enjoy being pregnant and described the birth as 'horrific'. When she was discharged from the hospital, she returned to live with Betty and Charles. For the first month, all was 'ok' and Jemma was at home caring for Teddy. She met her current partner when Teddy was one month old. She moved them both in with her partner after 4 weeks. Immediately there were concerns for Teddy.

Betty and Charles have encouraged Jemma to leave her partner, but she has refused. They were told by Jemma's partner they were not allowed to visit Teddy. When Jemma did bring him to their house, they could see Teddy was being neglected and not being fed properly. Betty and Charles offered to look after him which Jemma allowed on the 'odd occasion'. They decided to report Jemma to Social Services. Jemma and her partner were offered help but refused to engage.

Jemma has supervised contact with Teddy every other week, she sees him at Betty and Charles' home. She is inconsistent and when she does visit, she is disinterested in Teddy, preferring to watch TV. Teddy is very distressed when his mum visits and prefers to stay close to Betty. Jemma's partner drops her off and waits outside for up to 3 hours whilst she visits Teddy. She looks unkempt and is taking drugs. Betty and Charles would prefer not to have Jemma visit, they have made a request to Social Services for this to be reviewed with the possibility that contact is stopped. Their relationship with Jemma is strained and her two siblings will not speak to her. They do not like the way that she has treated their parents or Teddy.

Case Conceptualisation

Teddy has experienced early relational trauma and there is a high probability that he has witnessed domestic violence. Jemma's partner hates Teddy. She has alluded to the fact that he was violent towards Teddy when they were living together.

From Betty and Charles description and Teddy's presentation, it appears that he predominately moves into the mobilised state of sympathetic. It seems that he is co-regulated in the experience with Betty where he moves into ventral vagal. When Teddy was a baby, it appears that he dissociated in the presence of Jemma and her partner, moving into a protective dorsal state.

Betty and Charles are fully on board with any interventions offered to support Teddy. They are very angry with Jemma and are afraid for her well-being. They do not express their feelings to her, as the one time they did, her partner came into their house and punched Charles. They did not call the police for fear of reprisals.

Betty and Charles are aware that they are getting older and are concerned for Teddy's future.

Due to Teddy's presentation, it is felt that the most appropriate intervention would be Theraplay®. Betty and Charles will be offered therapeutic parenting and psychoeducation. Both know that they need personal therapy, Betty is open to this, Charles is not.

Tom

Age:	7 Years

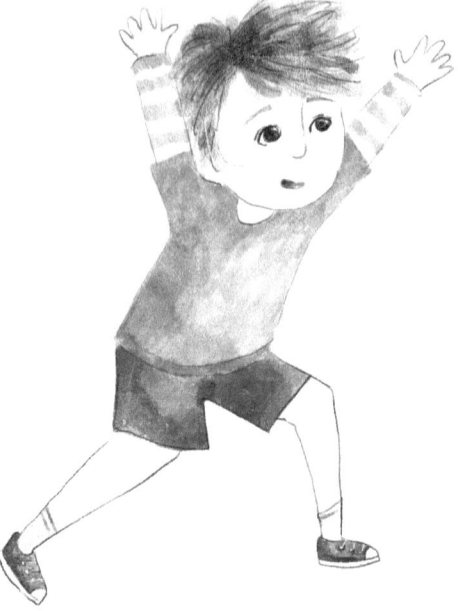

Figure 2.3 Tom.

Family Dynamics

Tom is the only child of Michelle and Paul who adopted him at 18 months. He was placed in foster care at 5 months old and remained with the same foster family until his adoption placement. Tom has not had contact with birth Mother or her extended family since the age of 13 months.

Developmental Milestones

Tom started walking at 10 months without ever crawling. It is reported that from the moment he could walk, he seemed to run everywhere. He is described as very clumsy, although he is a very able footballer. He hates lying on his tummy and struggles with some fine motor activities such as holding a pencil. All other developmental milestones were reported as being typical.

Additional Needs

Academically, Tom has additional support in the classroom and his school are seeking funding for him to have a one-to-one teaching assistant to support his social and emotional needs. He does not currently have a designated key worker but has developed a very strong relationship with his teacher. He has no diagnosed learning difference.

Medical History

Tom had an emergency delivery at 32 weeks by caesarean section. He remained in NICU for 5 days following his birth due to being underweight, needing oxygen support and jaundice prevention.

COVID-19 Experience

Tom had a mixed experience during the pandemic. He seemed to thrive having full parental attention during the initial lockdown when he stayed at home with both parents. However, he was unable to access online learning and would frequently 'fall apart' if any expectations were placed on him. His parents were able to get him back to school early and at this point his behaviours escalated. Tom would demonstrate dysregulated and challenging behaviours at home.

Reason for Referral

Tom was referred to therapy as both his parents and teachers find him very difficult to predict and manage. He has frequent meltdowns. For much of the time, neither his parents nor teachers can see the triggers which affect his family life and friendships at school. Michelle and Paul worry about taking him out of the home. They report that he is always on the move and is happiest when he is running around, climbing, or moving.

In school, Tom can have successful days. However, something will trigger him, and he will go back to hitting and kicking children or teachers with no warning. He does have friends, but the other children can be wary of him. He is not invited to playdates or birthday parties.

There are times Tom can cope at home. Michelle and Paul report that if he has their full attention, he seems happy, but they are exhausted as they cannot properly relax around him. They feel that Tom needs to process his early experiences and find ways to settle and calm down. Michelle and Paul have attempted to share Tom's life story with him. He won't engage fully and asks them to stop talking, becoming upset and angry if they persist. His behaviours are impacting family life as they can't go on holiday or family outings because as soon as he finds something stressful, he will act out, run away, or hit and kick.

Michelle, Paul, and the school are seeking support so Tom can develop self-regulation skills and process his early experiences. They would like Tom to be able to talk about how he feels so they can help him before he has a meltdown.

Background Information

Tom is a 7-year-old boy who was adopted by his parents Michelle and Paul at 18 months. He is their only child. His birth mother Sally was 18 years old and living in Supported Housing when Tom was born at 32 weeks. Sally had a very disrupted childhood and lived with multiple foster carers until she became pregnant at age 17.

During her pregnancy, Sally experienced high levels of stress due to domestic violence received from Tom's biological father. She rarely attended pregnancy checks and went into early labour which resulted in an emergency c-section. At birth Tom was placed in NICU for 5 days. Sally did not visit him. She was unable to exit her relationship with Tom's father and the violence towards her continued. Sally attempted to offer Tom care and love, but this was inconsistent. Whenever Tom's biological father would come to her property, she would protect him by placing him in his cot in a dark room.

At 5 months Tom was placed in foster care with Diane and Simon as it was determined that his needs were not being met. Tom had supervised contact with Sally until this broke down when he was 13 months old as she was not attending to him appropriately during visits. The foster carers described how Tom would cry and reach out for Sally. She always seemed very disengaged and would be looking at her phone or talking with friends during much of the time when visits were taking place.

When Tom went to live with Diane and Simon, they were caring for 2 siblings aged 4 and 6 years. Diane and Simon were highly experienced foster carers and got Tom into a routine quickly. They described how he was difficult to soothe and would frequently cry.

When Tom moved to live with Michelle and Paul, they noted that initially he was 'good as gold', playful and easy to settle. They described how after he had lived with them for three days it was like a switch went off. He couldn't tolerate routine, only falling asleep with both in the room. They found it very challenging to take him to playgroups or the park as he would frequently hit out at other children.

Michelle and Paul visited Tom at his foster carers a total of four times before he moved in to live with them. He initially had contact with his foster carers, but these visits stopped when Tom was 2.5 years old as Michelle and Paul felt it was too upsetting for him.

When Tom was aged 5 years, the family had Therapeutic Parenting Support to help them understand Tom's attachment history and to find strategies to help him settle. Michelle and Paul report that this intervention helped but they continue to struggle to understand Tom's behaviours. They describe that Tom is fine when he is with them, or when they can provide him with clear expectations and details of what is about to happen. However, he remains very unpredictable when in the 'outside' world and they continue to struggle to manage his aggressive responses as they cannot assess when he will have a meltdown.

Case Conceptualisation

Tom experienced developmental and relational trauma. He had a traumatic birth experience, was born prematurely and needed medical intervention. He received inconsistent, misattuned care during his first months of life and was left alone to self-regulate during frightening violent episodes in the home. By the age of 18 months, Tom had lived in three family settings. The caregivers he relied on all had different approaches to meeting his needs.

Michelle, Paul, and his teacher describe behaviours indicating a mobilised protective response. Tom flees and fights when feeling under threat. He can utilise the social engagement systems of both his parents and teachers, but is wholly reliant on their presence to remain in a regulated state.

Tom has not been able to process or integrate his early lived experience. Trauma was experienced during critical windows of development and will be stored as right-brain, bodily memories.

It is determined that alongside long-term individual Play Therapy, the therapist would have regular meetings with his parents and his teacher.

Hannah

Age:	9 Years Old

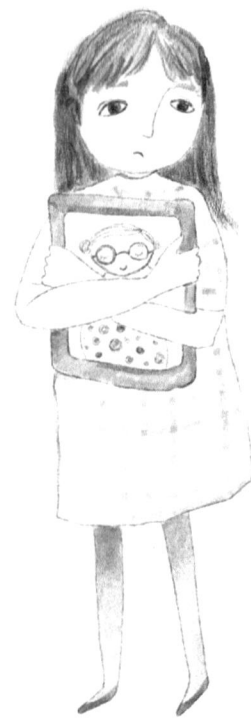

Figure 2.4 Hannah.

Family Dynamics

Hannah's parents are divorced. Hannah lives with her mother Claire and her older sister Lucy (11 years), she regularly sees her father, Mark.

Developmental Milestones

Hannah met all her milestones.

Additional Needs

None

Medical History

Hannah broke her arm when she was 7 years old falling off a swing. Otherwise, she is reported as a healthy child.

COVID-19 Experience

Hannah missed her friends and struggled to learn online. Her grandmother became ill during the latter pandemic period and so had to shield. This meant that Hannah was unable to have her usual cuddles or spend time with her grandmother which she found hard. She was able to travel between her parents' homes. Contact arrangements continued to try to mitigate too much change.

Reason for Referral

Hannah was referred to therapy by her mother at the age of 9 when her maternal grandmother died following a brief illness. Hannah was struggling to come to terms with her grandmother's death and was often tearful. She struggled to sleep on her own, needing Claire to stay with her until she fell asleep. Claire would typically find Hannah in her bed in the morning. She sought therapeutic support as she was finding it increasingly difficult to help Hannah through her grief whilst supporting her own widowed father and processing her own loss.

Background Information

Claire had a healthy pregnancy and delivered Hannah at 41 weeks in hospital. Hannah was 'an easy baby', slept well and was breastfed for the first 5 months of her life. Her mother was the primary caregiver throughout Hannah's early months. She returned to work when Hannah was 8 months old, wherein Hannah was cared for by her maternal grandparents.

Hannah's parents Mark and Claire divorced when Hannah was 3 years old. They started drifting apart when Hannah was 2.5 years. As the relationship became strained, they made the decision to separate. They continued to co-parent, providing consistency and shared values across the two households. Hannah's parents enjoy a good relationship, and they attend all family events together.

Developmentally, Hannah met all her milestones. Claire describes Hannah as sociable, popular and loves sports, adding "she fights with her sister about 50% of the time and then you can't keep them apart. They are the best of friends and worst of friends!!"

Case Conceptualisation

Information gathered through meeting Hannah's parents indicate that she has a secure attachment foundation and had her early needs met. She has consistently experienced co-regulation, attunement, healthy boundaries, and predictability.

Hannah comes from a loving home and her parents managed their separation well. Mark and Claire have supported Hannah through this difficult life-changing event well, ensuring that any ruptures experienced were repaired and addressed.

Hannah is struggling with the grief and loss associated with the death of her grandmother. She may also be processing feelings around missed opportunities of ongoing connection with her grandmother due to the pandemic. Whilst Hannah's grief is painful and pervasive, it is an appropriate response to the loss of an important adult in her life.

Mark and Claire are invested in supporting Hannah in the best way possible. Their intentions are to attend meetings to understand Hannah's response to her loss. The therapist believes that a strong alliance can be formed with both parents to ensure they can continue to support Hannah following the termination of therapy.

Hannah is offered 1:1 therapeutic support focused on supporting her to process her grief. It is likely that themes of loss and separation will emerge, with possible somatic reference to the separation of her parents when she was 3 years old. Alongside this, Mark and Claire will be supported to extend healing within the outside world, gaining a better understanding of Hannah's process and progress.

Emma

Age:	10 Years old

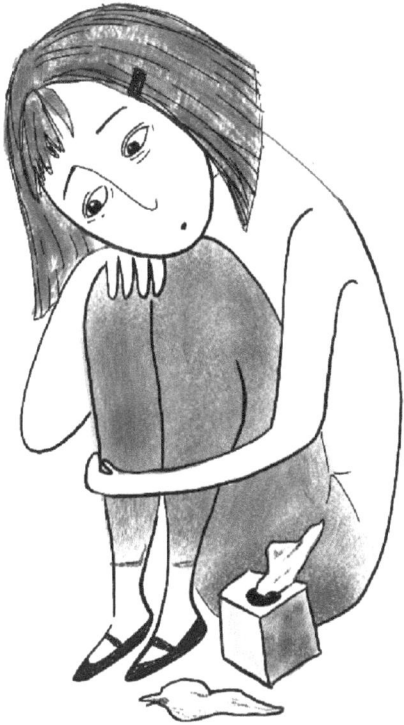

Figure 2.5 Emma.

Family Dynamics

Emma lives with her mother Dawn and her mother's partner Helen. Also in the home are Emma's siblings (16, 15, 13 years) and her stepsiblings (5 and 9 years). She has no contact with her father and hasn't seen him since she was 2 years old.

Developmental Milestones

Dawn reported that Emma met all her developmental milestones. During a meeting with Emma's school, they noted that Emma had few words at age 5 and needed Speech and Language Support.

Additional Needs

Following concerns from Emma's teacher about her social communication skills, resistance to change and preference for isolation, she had an assessment with an Educational Psychologist at age 7. It was confirmed that Emma did not meet the criteria for an Autistic Spectrum Diagnosis and does not have any specific learning difficulties, despite underachieving in all areas.

Medical History

Emma has enuresis and has attended multiple appointments with medical specialists to determine whether there are medical factors. To date they have concluded there is nothing physically wrong with her. Emma is still in pullups at night and frequently wets herself during the day but doesn't tell anyone. Emma is frequently ill and 'catches everything going'.

COVID-19 Experience

Dawn and Helen described their period in isolation as 'hell'. They were unable to support any of their children to engage in online learning as 'we don't have 5 computers'. The older children went back to school as soon as possible but they kept Emma and the younger one's home as 'they were no bother'. Helen has underlying health issues which meant that they were both really frightened of catching COVID-19. They describe how all the children seemed to go off the rails except for Emma who just kept to her usual quiet self.

Reason for Referral

Emma was referred to therapy by her school as they were concerned that she has few friends and is withdrawn and disengaged much of the time. She seems comfortable with one teaching assistant but doesn't talk to other staff members. Emma will not join in groups during break time or in the classroom.

Emma's teacher described her as 'slowly disappearing' and said that she knows nothing about her at all. She noted that Emma doesn't seem to have any likes, dislikes, or things she enjoys. She has a very poor attendance record due to frequent colds and stomach bugs.

The school's goals for therapy are for Emma to find at least one friend and smile. They would like her to be able to express her feelings and build relationships with the staff. They are very concerned about Emma's move to secondary school. They would also like her to know when she has wet herself.

The school have committed to providing funding for Emma to have therapeutic support for the 7 months whilst at primary school.

Background Information

Dawn left Emma's father when she was 7 months pregnant due to ongoing physical abuse towards herself and her older children. The family became a housing priority and were moved into a two-bedroom apartment. They have since moved homes three more times. Up until the age of 6 years, Emma slept in Dawn's room until Dawn met and moved in with Helen. Emma now shares a room with Helen's two younger children.

Dawn and Helen describe their household as very busy and chaotic. Social Services support the family due to ongoing challenges with Dawn's oldest two children (15 and 16 years) who can become aggressive and violent to other members of the family. Dawn doesn't perceive Social Services as being helpful and has a difficult relationship with her older children's school. This has been an ongoing point of tension and arguments for Dawn and Helen, who otherwise describe a loving and supporting relationship.

Dawn describes how she did her best to parent her 4 children. She was very grateful that Emma was the least demanding of her children, never making a fuss. Dawn describes Emma as always very quiet and as a good girl who helps around the house 'more than the other lot'.

Dawn and Helen note that they are very surprised that the school thinks Emma needs help as she is the least of their problems. When asked about Emma's strengths, they struggle to think about what she is good at, other than helping with their 5-year-old who she is reported to have the best relationship with.

Case Conceptualisation

Emma has witnessed domestic violence, insecure housing, unattuned parenting and ongoing sibling abuse. From interviews with school and her parents, it appears that Emma dissociates and spends much of her time in the protective dorsal state. She is underachieving in school and is unable to experience positive relationships. Emma has one tenuous relationship with a teaching assistant and is loving towards her youngest stepsiblings. She is unable to generalise this to other relationships.

It does not seem that Emma's parents have the capacity to fully involve themselves in the therapeutic process. Dawn and Helen have identified that they are both 'running around like idiots'. They will try to come to any meetings, but it would be easier to catch up on the phone. It is hoped that the therapist can support them to make the necessary changes needed to support Emma in the home.

Emma will be supported through 1:1 therapy. Consistent communication with teachers is necessary to help them support Emma's transition to her secondary school.

Ezra

Age:	10 Years old

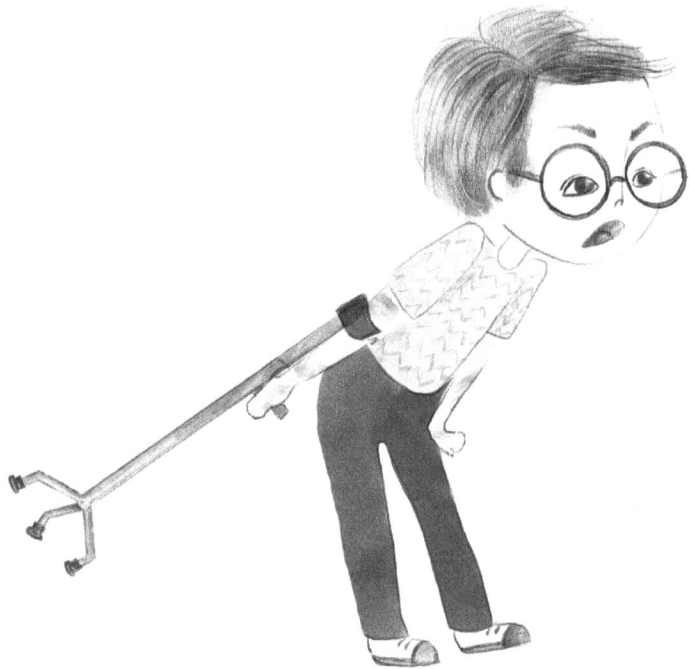

Figure 2.6 Ezra.

Family Dynamics

Ezra lives with Mum; Elizabeth, Dad; Jacob and Rachel, older sister aged 15 years. For the past ten years, Ezra's maternal grandparents have lived in a purpose-built annexe which is on the grounds of the property.

Developmental Milestones

Ezra has been slow to meet some of his developmental milestones as he has had many operations including skin grafting, releasing tendons due to sustaining 60% burns to his body.

Additional Needs

When Ezra was nearly two years old, he fell backwards into a bucket of boiling water. He suffered 60% burns to his body, not his face.

Medical History

Ezra has been under the care of the National Health Service due to a burn injury which he sustained as an infant.

COVID-19 Experience

Ezra was 9 years in COVID-19. He was deemed as vulnerable due to having skin grafting just before the first lockdown. Ezra's grandparents were also deemed vulnerable due to their own health needs.

Ezra's recovery was slow, and he was not well enough to attend school lessons online. Ezra was isolated and saw no friends throughout COVID-19. Elizabeth and Jacob reported that he became very 'clingy' in lockdown, describing him being like an 18 months old. Ezra's sleep has been terrible since his last operation. He often gets into his parent's bed and ends up sleeping next to Elizabeth. This has been a source of tension between his parents.

Elizabeth and Jacob have struggled caring for Ezra. There continues to be arguments between them as well as Elizabeth and her parents. Elizabeth and Jacob do not know if they will remain as a couple. They continue to live together, but Jacob is sleeping on the sofa every night. Ezra and Rachel often talk together and are worried that their parents will split up.

Reason for Referral

Ezra was referred for children and young person's counselling due concerns about regression and his struggles in engaging with peers. When in school, he is often tearful, goes to the medical room and requests to go home. Due to his trauma history, the school policy is that if Ezra is distressed for any reason, they contact home and generally it is one of his grandparents who collect him. Once back at home, Ezra shows no distress which is a source of irritation for Elizabeth and Jacob. In addition, when he feels overwhelmed at break times, he has permission to go to the school medical room until he feels better.

Ezra is not meeting attainment levels at school. He has no interest in any lessons other than art. He finds the classroom environment overwhelming and finds that he cannot move around easily as, he has walking sticks. When Ezra's movement is very bad, he uses his wheelchair. He can present as angry and has been known to throw his walking sticks when in the classroom. In these times, the teacher will evacuate the classroom and Ezra is left on his own. Nobody will enter the classroom until they see that Ezra has 'calmed down' which can sometimes take up to 2 hours.

Background Information

Ezra was born full term and was a much-wanted baby. Elizabeth and Jacob are medics and in the armed forces. They are often away on tour, sometimes at the same time, sometimes at different times. When Ezra was about one year, Elizabeth, and Jacob along with her parents decided to purchase a larger house with an annexe to live together. Elizabeth and Jacob felt that this would offer consistency for the children and help with any childcare issues as Elizabeth's parents could look after Rachel and Ezra.

Just before Ezra's second birthday, Elizabeth and Jacob were on tour. Ezra was in the care of Elizabeth's parents. It was winter, the boiler was broken and there was no heating or hot water. Ezra's grandparents were waiting for a heating engineer to sort and in the meantime had been boiling kettles for hot water. This night, Elizabeth's Mum filled a bucket with water so the children could have a bath. The bucket was in the bathroom. She left the bathroom to get towels, seconds later she heard Ezra screaming to find him sat in the bucket. He was flown to the nearest burns unit, his parents were contacted and returned from the tour. Ezra has had more than 50 operations since aged two years and will continue to have. He has 60% burns to all parts of his body other than his face. He has toes and fingers amputated. His mobility on many levels is limited.

Case Conceptualisation

Ezra suffered a big T physical trauma before his second birthday. He continues to suffer physically, emotionally, and psychologically. The circumstances of Ezra's burn injury and amputations have caused distress and arguments between all family members. Elizabeth and Jacob blame her parents. During COVID-19 this caused a lot more tension between them all. In one heated argument, Elizabeth and Jacob shouted out that they hated her parents for what they had done. That they had ruined the family.

Ezra finds it difficult to move into the ventral vagal at school other than when he is in the company of the school nurse. He feels safe in the medical room and is happy to chat with the nurse about anything and everything. All other times at school, he moves between sympathetic and dorsal vagal. However, he tends to move towards sympathetic arousal. At home, Ezra also moves between sympathetic and dorsal vagal states, especially in the presence of his parents. At night-time, he seeks comfort from his mum. From a hierarchy perspective Ezra is seeking connection; ventral vagal. Mostly, Ezra is calm in the presence of his grandparents which shows that he is leaning towards cues of safety rather than cues of danger. When these cues change, he moves towards sympathetic and mobilisation, crying and screaming. Ezra would benefit from a trauma-focused intervention, The Needs Paradox© for children and The Needs Paradox© for parent-child dyads. It would also be beneficial for Elizabeth and Jacob to access couple counselling as well as family therapy for everyone. It is worth noting, that Rachel leans towards dorsal. Ezra continues to have treatment under the NHS for his burn injury.

Chapter 3

Internal Surveillance System

The Polyvagal Theory provides therapists working with children with a neuro-physiological framework to consider the reasons why children act in the ways that they do. It provides us with a neurobiological answer as to why children experience positive and negative reactions or behaviours whilst interacting with others. Responses to the environment happen autonomically, which means it is an involuntary process. Many behaviours we see are generated by the autonomic nervous system well below the level of conscious awareness. Through this framework we come to understand that the behaviours that bring children into the therapy room are involuntary energies moving in patterns of protection. The brain is not making a cognitive choice to react but rather reactions happen to children.

The Polyvagal Theory is hugely hopeful and demonstrates that whilst early experiences shape the nervous system, ongoing experiences can reshape it. Just as the brain is continually changing in response to experiences and the environment, our autonomic nervous system is likewise engaged and can be intentionally influenced (Dana, 2018). It is imperative that therapists understand that feeling safe is a biological process which is supported by regulating relationships with others. We, as therapists, are in the perfect position to offer our clients a felt sense of safety, which will allow them to move into a more regulated, social engagement system.

In this chapter, we start by outlining the anatomy of the nervous system. This is essential to our understanding, as it moves us to consider behaviours and responses from a body-based, biological lens; rather than a cognitive one. Once we grasp the notion that children in our therapy rooms are involuntarily responding to information provided to them on a body-based level, shame and judgement is removed, paving the way for self-compassion and self-understanding.

We then introduce you to the Social Engagement System, the newest neural circuit which has developed to promote mammalian survival through connection, social bonds and signals of safety. It is through our social engagement system that we can develop relationships, learn, play and be an active part of our community.

DOI: 10.4324/9781003412571-4

It is the core of humanness, necessary for our survival and is often the part of the nervous system which is least familiar to the clients we work with.

Finally, we explain the three organising principles of the Polyvagal Theory:

- Neuroception: the process by which our Autonomic Nervous System detects cues of safety and threat without awareness. The Autonomic Nervous System seeks information from three sources: Internally (inside the body); Environmentally (outside the body) and in Interaction (with people). In the face of threat there are three possible outcomes:

  1 remain in engagement (connection)
  2 become mobilised (fight/flight)
  3 become immobilised (collapse)

- Hierarchy: explains how the three possible outcomes to a neuroception of threat occur in a hierarchical manner, according to the energy required to defend oneself.
- Co-regulation: the essential ingredient in supporting our clients to experience cues of safety and move away from involuntary protective responses. Co-regulation is a connection between two nervous systems whereby reciprocal regulation of autonomic states takes place. Essentially, we are lending our nervous system (Dion, 2021) to our clients, providing them with an experience of a regulated state and supporting them to develop this capacity for themselves.

The Nervous System

The nervous system is a network of neurons and nerve fibres which exist to transmit information throughout our body through electrical impulses. The core job of the nervous system is to provide us with information from our surrounding environment so we can respond to it. The nervous system has two divisions:

- The Central Nervous System (CNS) which is made up by the brain and the spinal cord
- The Peripheral Nervous System (PNS) consisting of nerves which branch out from the brain and spinal cord

Within the PNS there are two nerve types, the spinal nerves (pairs or bundles of nerves which emerge from the spinal cord) and the cranial nerves (nerves which emerge directly from within the brain). The PNS has two divisions. The Somatic Nervous System which is known as the voluntary nervous system and carries motor and sensory signals to the brain and, the Autonomic Nervous System (ANS) which is known as the involuntary nervous system. Figure 3.1 provides a map of the nervous system.

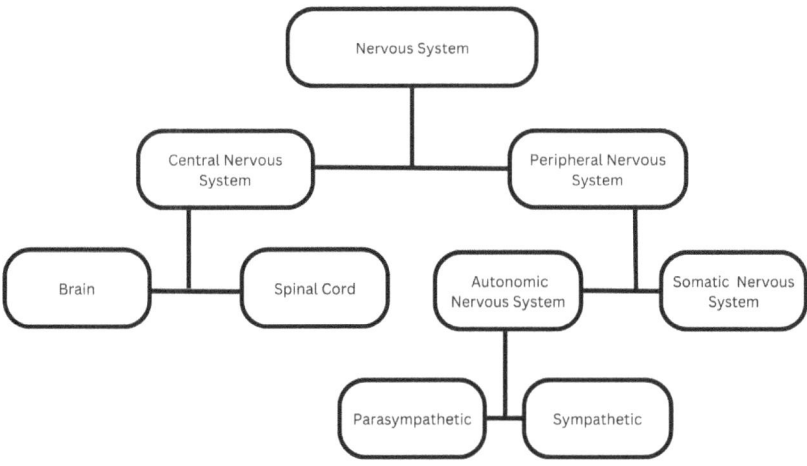

Figure 3.1 Nervous system map.

The Autonomic Nervous System (ANS)

The ANS continuously works to oversee all involuntary autonomic functions needed to stay alive. The ANS is divided into the parasympathetic nervous system and the sympathetic nervous system. Both systems control the same bodily functions but with opposite effects and it is their job to work together to maintain balance, encouraging stability within the body. The sympathetic nervous system instigates energy in the body, preparing it for activity. In contrast, the parasympathetic nervous system does the exact opposite, slowing things down and inhibiting high-energy functions.

The table in Figure 3.2 identifies some of the physiological functions of both branches and shows us how important it is that these two systems work together.

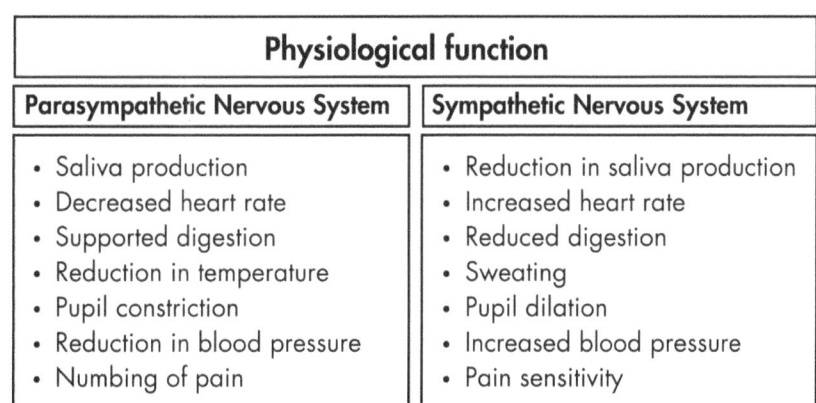

Figure 3.2 Physiological function.

Too much emphasis on one division can have a marked impact on physiological outcomes and the balance of the body system.

The Vagus Nerve

Within the ANS are 31 spinal nerves and 12 cranial nerves, creating a network which allows the body to always function on an unconscious level. The Polyvagal Theory is focused on the work of the vagus nerve which is the 10th cranial nerve. As the longest cranial nerve and starting in the brain, the vagus nerve wanders through the face, thorax, chest, abdomen, and gut relaying information from every organ back to the brain. Figure 3.3 offers an illustration of the vagus nerve.

The vagus nerve lies within the parasympathetic nervous system and is considered one of its main components. Its core job is to regulate and support the return to homeostasis of all our internal organs. It sends bidirectional communication between the gut and the brain, modulating the heart rate, respiratory rate, temperature, and digestion, influencing the following:

- our immune system
- speech
- sleep
- vomiting
- sneezing
- swallowing
- toileting

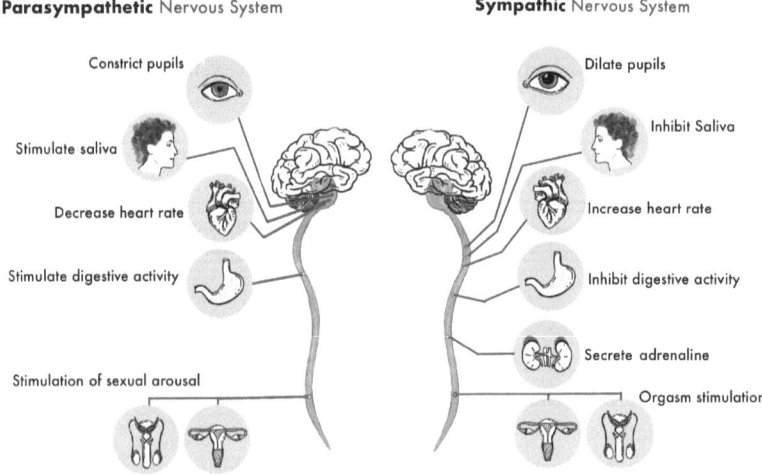

Figure 3.3 The vagus nerve.

Often thought of as a superhighway, the vagus nerve processes information from the body to the brain constantly, without awareness. When the vagus nerve is stimulated it elicits a response from the parasympathetic nervous system which then balances energy and output, causing a reduction of sympathetic activation and a return to homeostasis.

Introducing the Ventral Vagal System

Through his introduction of the Polyvagal Theory, Porges proposes that the parasympathetic vagus nerve has two branches, the Ventral Vagal System and the Dorsal Vagal System which originate in the same area of the brain (medulla oblongata). The Ventral Vagal System sits above the diaphragm, the Dorsal Vagal is located below the diaphragm and into the gut. Whilst the Dorsal Vagal System is found in reptiles, mammals, and birds, the Ventral Vagal System is found only in mammals and has evolved very specifically to encourage social engagement and connection.

The Ventral Vagal System is also referred to as the Social Engagement System. Whilst the Social Engagement System is myelinated, allowing information to travel through the nerve at a speedier rate, the Dorsal Vagal System is unmyelinated which means it is much slower at sending electrical impulses to the brain. Another way of thinking about this is the social engagement branch of the vagus nerve is like a high-speed broadband connection. You can download data, send, and receive emails immediately, make video calls and rely on it to do what you need it to do. The dorsal vagal branch is dial-up. It is a slow processing system, needs to whir around to connect, trying to find the link and takes a whilst to send and receive information. Figure 3.4 shows the Polyvagal understanding of the Autonomic Nervous System.

Reconsidering the physiological functions of the ANS with the inclusion of the Social Engagement System (Ventral Vagal Complex) we can see that the body is not consistently hanging in the balance of too much or not enough energy. This third system provides opportunities for us to be in homeostasis and have access to all brain regions, whilst seeking connection with others. Please see Figure 3.5 for a reconsideration of the physiological functions of the ANS.

Through Porges' introduction to the concept of the Social Engagement System, the vagus nerve's influence on the ANS is not limited to 'stop' and 'go'. There is a third option of 'connect' and it is through the introduction of this concept that interest in the ANS shifts from being exclusively related to physical regulation, to affect regulation and a felt sense of safety.

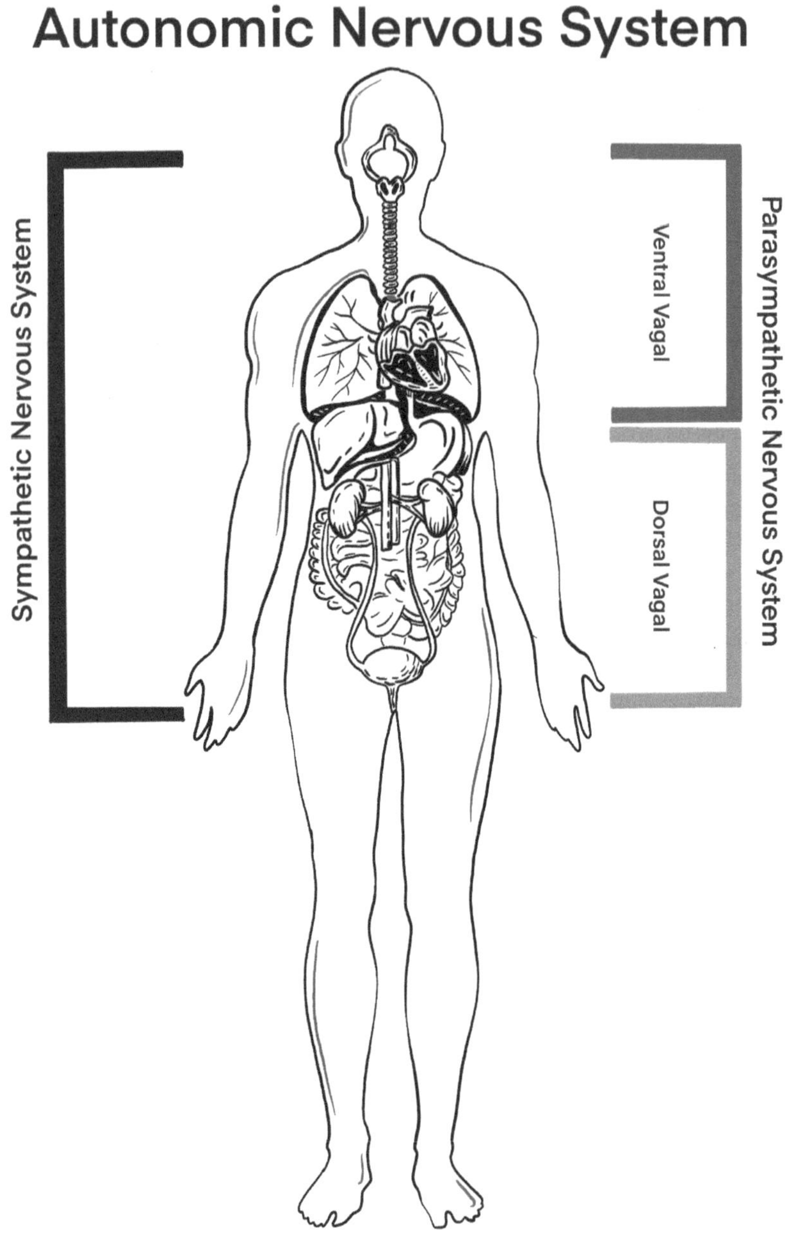

Autonomic Nervous System

Sympathetic Nervous System

Ventral Vagal

Dorsal Vagal

Parasympathetic Nervous System

Figure 3.4 The Autonomic Nervous System.

Physiological function		
Ventral Vagal Complex	**Sympathetic Nervous System**	**Dorsal Vagal Complex**
• Steady heart rate • Healthy metabolism • Average temperature • Diaphragmatic breath • Steady blood pressure • Maintain eye contact	• Reduction in saliva production • Increased heart rate • Reduced digestion • Sweating • Quick shallow breath • Pupil dilation • Increased blood pressure • Pain sensitivity	• Saliva production • Decreased heart rate • Supported digestion • Reduction in temperature • Slow breath • Pupil constriction • Reduction in blood pressure • Numbing of pain

Figure 3.5 Physiological function and the Ventral Vagal Complex.

The Social Engagement System

The Social Engagement System (Ventral Vagal System) is the branch of the parasympathetic nervous system which affects body functioning above the diaphragm. It connects our facial muscles to our heart and lungs, sending out signals of safety and seeking relationship. The Social Engagement System requires a felt sense of safety. In these conditions, it supports us to interact with other social engagement systems, have relationships and develop social bonds. When we are in our Social Engagement System, signals of safety are sent to other nervous systems by utilising gentle prosody and easy eye gaze. Generalised sound is filtered out and we are able to focus in on the human voice.

In 1975, Ed Tronick presented his findings from The Still Face experiment. The experiment begins with a parent and baby facing each other. The parent smiles and plays with the baby utilising their social engagement system. They then turn away and look back at the baby with no expression and lack of responsiveness. The parent has intentionally switched off their social engagement system. The baby makes repeated attempts to reengage the parent, first by smiling and making gentle sounds, when this fails to elicit a positive reaction, the baby quickly becomes dysregulated. The findings were hugely influential on Modern Attachment Theory and demonstrate how babies will work very hard to achieve face-to-face connection with their caregiver. When the connection is denied and the baby is presented with a flat face 'still face', there is an immediate impact on the baby physiologically and emotionally. This experiment shows how greatly we rely on the Social Engagement System for connection and when this is unavailable, our nervous system becomes dysregulated as it cannot find a sense of safety.

Therapists utilise their social engagement system. Through the heart-to-face connection, we seek non-verbal cues and empathically respond, focus on hearing our client's voices and change in tone, as well as using facial cues and gentle prosody to elicit a neuroception of safety.

The Internal Surveillance System: Neuroception

Imagine you have a silent, highly qualified, rigorous Super Protector© inside your body. The Super Protector's job is to scan for safety or danger constantly, ensuring that you are ready to respond to any perceived threat within a millisecond without you ever having to think about it. The technical term for this Super Protector© is neuroception.

Porges (2003, 2004) gave us the term neuroception to describe the unconscious process of reading cues and assessing the need to respond to signals of danger. Neuroception surveils in three areas: in the environment, inside the body, and in response to other nervous systems. If threat is detected in any of those areas, three potential autonomic outcomes occur:

1 You stay connected to yourself and seek connection in others. The threat is not unmanageable, you can think, talk, communicate, and remain socially engaged. You are in the Ventral Vagal System. We refer to this as the AWAKE STATE.

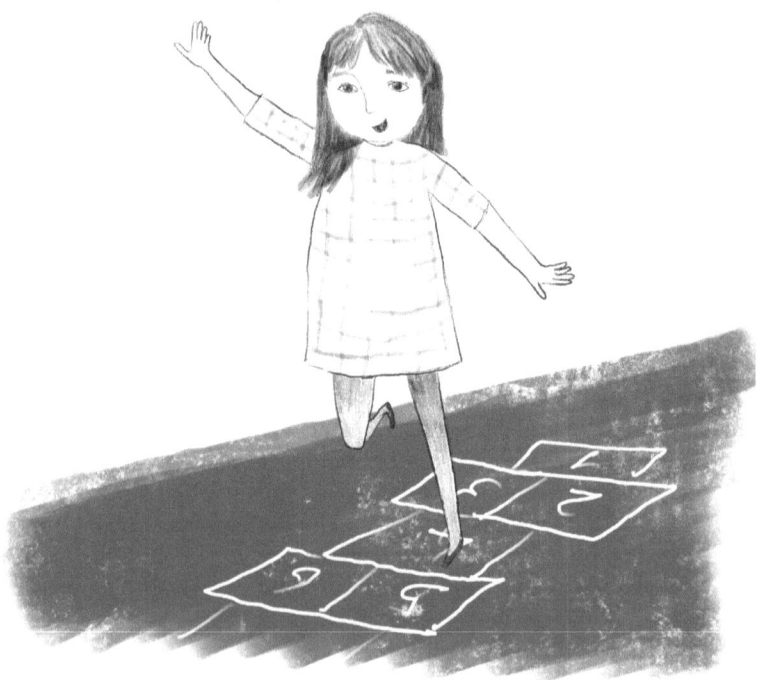

Figure 3.6 Hannah in the AWAKE State.

2 You need to do something. The threat is such that you need to act which is often referred to as the fight flight response. You are sympathetically activated. We refer to this as the ALARM STATE.

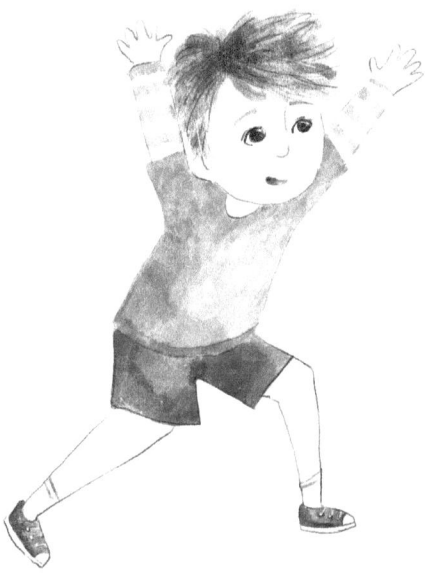

Figure 3.7 Tom in the ALARM State.

3 You need to hide. Doing something is not going to help. You've gone quiet, numbed, collapsed. You are in the Dorsal Vagal System. We refer to this as the AVOID STATE.

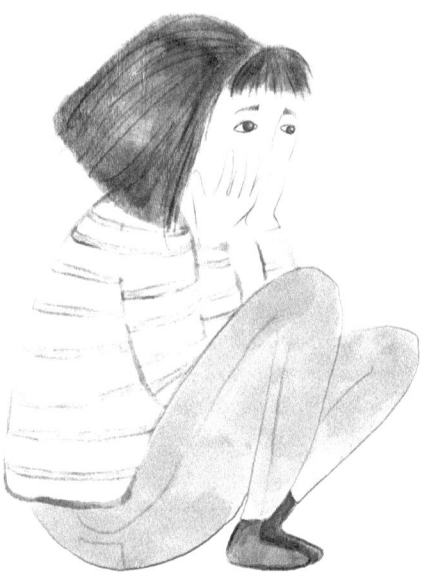

Figure 3.8 Emma in the AVOID State.

Let's imagine you are standing in a school playground and a group of 30 children are on their mid-morning break, it is a sunny day and there are two teachers on duty keeping an eye on the children as they enjoy some free time. There is a general sound of laughter, some playful shouting and a lot of movement as children dart around quickly from place to place. Hannah is sitting on a bench talking and playing hand clapping games with a friend. You can assume that Hannah is in her Ventral Vagal System. She is, chatting, connecting, moving in and out of eye contact and smiling at friends. Another group of children are playing football, and they accidentally kick the football so it careers towards Hannah causing her to jump away, scream and then burst out laughing. No one was hurt and whilst she initially and autonomically moved into flight, neuroception quickly determined that she was no longer in threat. She returned to social connection and resumed her game. Hannah is in the AWAKE STATE.

A minute later, the teacher shouts "Tom no! Do not hit Joe!" and runs towards the group of footballers. You turn to see Tom fleeing from his footballing friends, heading towards the school gate. As the teacher reaches Tom, he kicks out at her, his eyes are like darts, and it seems like he is defending himself against a terrifying predator. The teacher gives him space, holds out her hands and bends down showing Tom she means no harm. Eventually he moves towards her and together they leave the playground. During a later conversation with the teacher, she shares that Tom often has 'meltdowns' and hits out at other children, "It happens for no reason. It's such a shame because he is doing so well a lot of the time." Could it be that Tom experiences a neuroception of danger when his heartrate and temperature arrive at the same levels as when he was a toddler hiding from his dad? Tom is in the ALARM STATE.

You then notice Emma sitting in the corner of the playground, she seems oblivious to the commotion around her. Her body is slumped, she has no facial affect seeming almost to be asleep, and she is twirling her hair around her finger with an empty gaze. One of the teachers approaches her and attempts to engage her in conversation. The teacher reaches out her hand and it seems to you that she is encouraging Emma to move. Her facial expression doesn't change, and she remains still, appearing not to hear her teacher's words. Based on this interaction, you consider whether Emma's system is overwhelmed with the chaos, inconsistency and noise. She seems to be shutdown, without energy or "spark" (Music, 2022). Emma is in the AVOID STATE.

We can see from the above vignettes three very different responses in the same environment. Hannah was in the AWAKE State. She was laughing, playing relatively complex games, and responded to the threat of the football by leaping out the way temporarily moving into sympathetic activation. Her ALARM State was quickly inhibited, and she returned to social engagement as soon as the threat had passed.

Tom appeared socially engaged, running with his friends, and taking part in a mutual game. As his heart rate and temperature increased, a neuroception of threat instigated a sympathetic response and he moved into the fight flight activation. Tom was in the ALARM State. He attempted to fight his way out of danger and run away from the perceived threat. Tom was unable to read the facial cues of his teacher, he tuned out her voice so he could listen out for "sounds of danger" (Dana, 2018, p. 25) and continued to defend himself in a mobilised and activated way.

Emma was overwhelmed by the environment. Her system downregulated, she became hypo aroused and was in deep protection, shutting down all connection with the outside world, she was in the AVOID State. The environment presented a neuroception of extreme threat moving her into dorsal immobilisation, "the path of last resort" (Dana, 2018, p. 23). She became truly alone in her experience.

Hannah, Tom, and Emma's behaviours take place autonomically, without thought or consideration. The playground is familiar to all the children, with two teachers on duty meeting their needs, ready to help and offer support and kindness. As the observer there doesn't appear to be an obvious threat. Why then do some children feel unsafe in an environment that is safe? Porges (2015, 2017) notes that feeling safe not only requires the absence of threat, but also the presence of safety cues discernible to the nervous system.

The Development of Neuroception

If a child is raised in a safe, nurturing, responsive environment, they will experience a consistent neuroception of safety on a neurobiological level. Their systems are ready to respond to perceptions of threat appropriately and return to homeostasis easily as their generalised expectation is that the world is safe. If a child is raised in an environment where there is a neuroception of threat, their system is primed to always respond to danger and does so regardless of whether the threat is present in the here and now. They have limited access to safe and social connection, instead are ready to defend to survive. According to Porges (2011), "People with impaired social engagement systems are prone to misinterpret safety as a threat and objective dangers as safety".

Think of a smoke alarm in your kitchen at home. The batteries are working, and the smoke alarm has only ever sounded once when you forgot to take food out of the oven and smoke was pouring out. Called to action, you open the window, pressed the reset button, and probably threw out the food! Calm was resumed and the smoke alarm was ready for the next cooking disaster.

Now imagine there is a faulty wire in the smoke alarm, and it goes off all the time. Whether you are making toast, opening the oven door, blowing out a match, the alarm sounds! This smoke alarm has a mind of its own. You must wait for the engineer to fix the alarm just in case there is a real fire, and you have no choice but to rely on the faulty system until it is repaired.

Let's imagine Hannah enjoys a functional smoke alarm. She is familiar with the AWAKE State. Her system responds appropriately to threat, and she can return to a safe and social position once the threat has passed.

Often referred to as Adaptive Neuroception, we prefer to borrow the term Matched Neuroception from Deb Dana, wherein the response to threat is appropriate, it matches the situation bringing in enough energy as required to defend against the presenting situation.

Now, let's imagine Emma and Tom who have smoke alarms which need attention. They have mismatched neuroception. Their ANS' have developed in service of protection which interferes with their ability to neurocept safety, causing them to tumble into responses which were of service to them in the past. Emma disappears into the AVOID State and Tom flees to the ALARM State.

At one time these responses matched. It was adaptive and necessary for their autonomic nervous systems to protect them in this way, and they survived as a result. Their nervous systems have not had enough exposure to safety cues and as a result they rely on historical, unconscious responses to defend themselves.

Moving between States: Hierarchy

Porges refers to the Polyvagal Theory as "the Science of Safety" (2022). He considers "our need to feel safe as a biological imperative linked to survival" (2022) and how safe we feel is directly linked to data and information produced from within the body. The moment our ANS moves us out of the Ventral Vagal System, we lose capacity for connection and become primed for protection. We either do something, or if the threat is big enough or life-threatening, we collapse.

The Polyvagal Theory determines that our responses to threat occur in a hierarchical manner. We can only move from the AWAKE State to the AVOID State, having first experienced a measure of ALARM. Likewise, to return to the connected AWAKE State from the collapsed AVOID State, we must mobilise ourselves through the activated ALARM State. Deb Dana (2018) conceptualises hierarchy as a ladder offering a visual map which supports consideration of each of the three autonomic states: Ventral Vagal, Sympathetic and Dorsal Vagal as an up and down movement, mirroring the anatomical branches of the vagus nerve. We represent this concept below through ANS 'A' States, in a triangular formation illustrating the movement between protective responses alongside the neural capacity for openness and connection.

ANS 'A' States

The ANS 'A' States are illustrated in Figure 3.9.

In the AWAKE State, there is capacity to migrate through the brainstem and have access to all brain regions. This allows us to be present in the moment, engage in learning, have conversations, play, and seek connection. Communication between the right and left hemispheres is possible. Our brain is in charge, encouraging us to make the most of the here and now and respond appropriately to our environment.

The ALARM State has a solid relationship with the limbic system, particularly the amygdala and the hypothalamus. The adrenal glands get busy and pump adrenaline into the bloodstream and the body is mobilised. In this State our executive functioning is compromised, and we are largely hostage to our 'emotional brain' making decisions for us.

In the AVOID State we only have access to the brain stem which is wholly in service of survival. There is no capacity for thought. Fundamentally, we share the same brain capacity as reptiles and birds responding to our environment as if danger is everywhere.

It is proposed (Porges & Furman, 2011) that the concept of hierarchy is phylogenetic, which means the mammalian autonomic nervous system has developed according to evolutionary necessity. As mammals there was a survival need to prioritise social communication, social bonds and the establishment of safe environments.

Humans are always looking for safety, as such, in the face of threat we will first turn to the AWAKE State which is the newest evolutionary circuit. This system works hard to seek connection with another nervous system and inhibiting the need to fight or run. It is only if there is a neuroception of danger that older circuits are recruited, first turning to our ALARM State and then finally to the

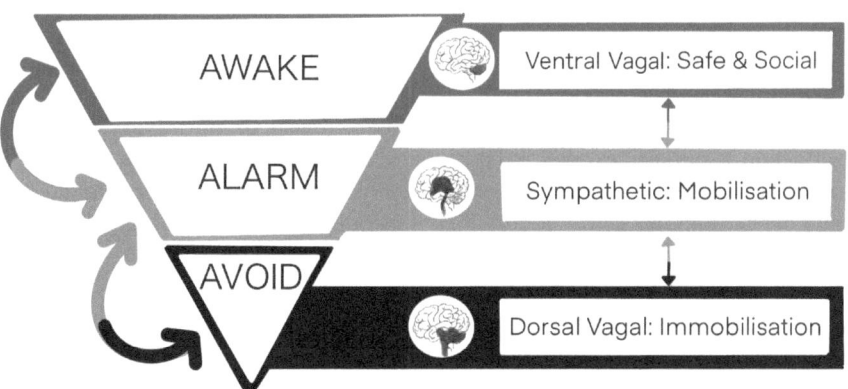

Figure 3.9 ANS 'A' States.

AVOID State if necessary. The Polyvagal Theory considers that the development of the Social Engagement System was necessary to ensure the survival of connection-needing mammals, as, "To survive mammals must determine friend from foe, when an environment is safe, and communicate to their social unit" (Porges, 2009).

In order to return to the AWAKE State from either of the two protective states, the "mammalian nervous system needs to perform two important adaptive tasks: (1) assess risk, and (2) if the environment is perceived a safe, inhibit the more primitive limbic structures that control fight, flight, or freeze behaviours" (Porges, 2009).

Peter Levine developed Somatic Experiencing® after spending years studying how animals recover themselves following severe trauma. When chased by a predator, a preyed upon mammal will first attempt to get away and then feign death in an attempt to trick their predator into pretending they are dead. Once the threat is removed the animal will start to shake and tremble with an eventual return to homeostasis, as if the event never took place. In the face of threat, the animal moved from the AWAKE State into the ALARM State then onto the AVOID State as a last resort. In order to re-emerge from the AVOID State the animal moved its body, elevating its heart rate which supported a return to the AWAKE State.

A return from the AVOID State is particularly challenging as this requires movement from the slower more stubborn dial-up (unmyelinated) system through activation. Graham Music (2022) reminds us of the biological precedent for halting energy production in the face of threat, "When our mitochondria … sense a threat, they shut down energy production and signal danger, so that much communication within the body between cells and organs stops" (p. 19). In all cases, when neurobiological shutdown occurs, a reboot is required to encourage the return of energy, this cannot happen until the perception of threat has passed. Signals of safety must be experienced and reexperienced to override the extreme danger signals that instigated immobilisation. We are asking children whose smoke alarm is faulty, to trust us enough that a change in battery is the safer and healthier option. This is a big ask!

We must emphasise that all three states perform valuable functions other than offering us protective responses to threat. We will need to move into sympathetic activation to run, feel excited and overcome challenge. To sleep, meditate or enjoy back-to-back box sets under a duvet, our nervous systems are required to move us into dorsal immobilisation. Figure 3.10 illustrates the hierarchical functional purpose and protective response of each state:

It is also important to remember that no one state is preferable. Each state is worthy, performative and necessary. We will be moving through these states throughout the day according to moment-by-moment interactions with the environment. Our bodies are designed to respond to external stimuli with appropriate energy. We are not designed to remain in any one protective state for long periods of time. A healthy autonomic nervous system is able to utilise the 'vagal brake'

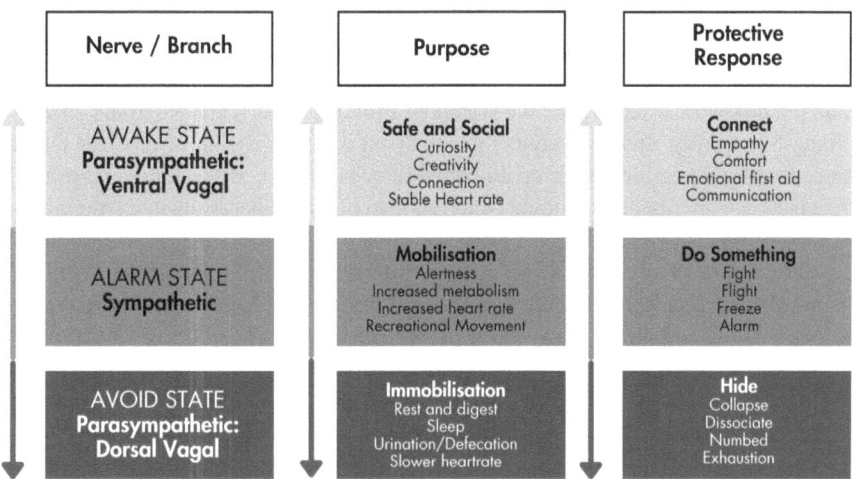

Figure 3.10 Hierarchical responses.

to stabilise the heart rate and return the system back to the AWAKE State, ready for connection.

> *Let's consider Amira and her ANS 'A' States. During Amira's time in NICU, and when resting in Layla's arms, all her vital signs are stable. Amira is being co-regulated by Layla; she is the AWAKE State. When Amira is placed back into the incubator, her heart rate increases, and she begins to flail. She is in sympathetic activation and in the ALARM State. Finally, Amira goes into collapse as she is metabolically depleted which is due to the cost of high sympathetic arousal. Amira is in the AVOID State.*

The Vagal Brake

When we are ventral vagally mediated (in the AWAKE State) it positively influences our heart rate, acting like a pacemaker and ensuring that it beats rhythmically according to the need at the time. This process is referred to as the vagal brake, without it our heart would beat dangerously fast. The vagal brake supports us to move into experiencing challenge whilst remaining in the AWAKE State. You can run, play, get excited, watch a horror film, all without tipping into the fight flight response. The vagal brake gives us enough energy and an increase in activation without pushing us into a felt sense of danger which would cause the release of cortisol and adrenaline, resulting in full activation of the ALARM State. According to Porges, "Functionally, the vagal brake, by modulating visceral state, enables the individual to rapidly engage and disengage with objects and other individuals and to promote self-soothing behaviours and calm states" (2007).

At its most efficient, the vagal brake gently releases and inhibits according to the challenge, whilst remaining in the AWAKE State; this is self-regulation. If the vagal brake releases too quickly it stops the ventral vagal flow influencing the heart and pushes us into activation. We are taken from the AWAKE State to the ALARM State. Sometimes this is of course necessary if a neuroception of threat is experienced and we need to move or do something. However, when the vagal brake is released, we are unable to connect and relate to others, this results in dysregulation.

Let's relate this to Tom and Emma's experiences in the playground. Initially, whilst playing football Tom's vagal brake was relaxed and providing his system with enough energy so he could run and remain socially adaptive whilst experiencing a raised heartrate and increase in temperature.

Our hypothesis is that a neuroception of danger was elicited as a result of changes to his internal state, wherein his vagal brake released moving him into the ALARM State. Thinking about, Emma we can see that her vagal brake had released completely. Her neuroception of threat was so frightening that her capacity for social engagement was completely removed and had become the threat itself. Her system had collapsed and shutdown, the AVOID State, as identified by her flat facial affect, sleepy eyelids and lack of awareness of the sound of her teacher's voice.

Vagal Tone

Vagal Tone describes the activity of the vagus nerve and can be measured indirectly by heart rate variability. When vagal tone is high, the vagal brake acts as a pacemaker. Heart rate can increase but continues to be influenced by the Social Engagement System, so we are not moved into protecting ourselves. Children with high vagal tone can play sword fighting or engage in rough play without spilling into needing to fight to survive. Their bodies have cues of safety which informs them they are playing. With a high vagal tone, the vagal brake only releases completely if mobilisation is necessary, for example if something frightening happens and you need to fight or flee. With a low vagal tone, the vagal brake is unable to distinguish real threat from perceived resulting in a faulty smoke alarm.

Hannah's vagal brake released just enough energy to activate her to jump away from the football. Having high vagal tone, she quickly moved back into the socially engaged AWAKE State, resuming connection and returning to full brain functioning. Tom and Emma have low vagal tone, with weakened vagal brakes. They both experience mismatched neuroception with highly charged Super Protectors© who are focused on defence and survival.

Positive therapeutic intervention supports the strengthening of vagal tone, resulting in an effective vagal brake. This supports the Super Protector© to do its job optimally by assessing for safety and threat. This process occurs through the reciprocal sending and receiving of signals of safety from one nervous system to another and comprises the third organising principle of the Polyvagal Theory: Co-regulation.

Co-regulation

According to Polyvagal Theory, co-regulation is the connection between two nervous systems, each regulating the other in the process. For human beings to survive they need to form social bonds and have social communication. It is a biological imperative to seek interpersonal connection. The Polyvagal Theory provides a neurobiological framework within which we can consider the biological need for connection.

From the earliest days of psychoanalytical theory, we have understood that having an attuned relationship during early development offers the best chances of living a healthy and adaptive life. In 1966, D.W. Winnicott stated "There is no such thing as a baby, there is a baby and someone", capturing the importance of the primary caregiver's psychic functioning in the development of the infant's psychological processes. At birth, infants have access to their socially engaged AWAKE State, so that they can signal their needs to their caregiver by crying, smiling or shrieking (Porges, 2004). Through this process, the infant is utilising its social

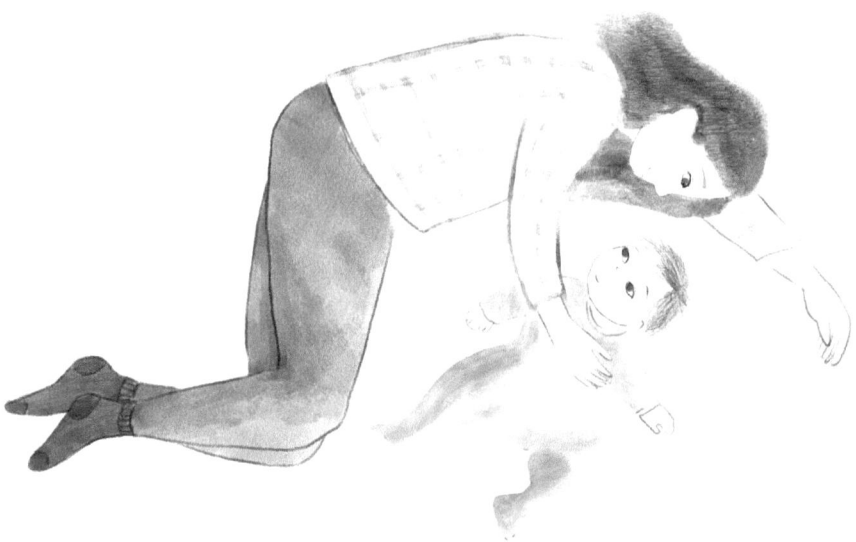

Figure 3.11 Co-regulation.

engagement system to connect with the adult on whom it so deeply relies. As these needs are met, the infant and caregiver co-regulate autonomic states via reciprocal cues of safety (Porges, 2022).

Returning to Amira, when we consider the traumatic birth, we see that both Layla's and Amira's nervous systems would have been under stress. Neither had the benefits of skin to skin contact as Amira was transferred to NICU after birth. Layla's physiology was not able to offer autonomic safety cues and connectedness. There was no opportunity for Layla to use her own heartbeat and breathing to stabilise Amira's heart rate and regulate her heartbeat through co-regulation.

The Polyvagal Theory provides us with a biological understanding of what has long been understood, with "overwhelming empirical support for the fact that early experience is a powerful force in development" (Siegel and Sroufe, 2011). An attuned caregiver provides nurture and soothes the infant as they move through different states of arousal. A crying baby is attended to and rocked. A smiling baby is smiled back at sending signals of a joined experience. A cooing baby is spoken to with gentle prosody (Kolacz *et al.*, 2021). The Social Engagement System is at work (eyes, voice, facial muscles) as the primary caregiver utilises their Ventral Vagal System to offer consistency and care to the infant, which in turn leads the infant to experience unity (Winnicott, 1966) and co-regulation. Through being nurtured and soothed, infants' neural pathways are strengthened leading to the development of high vagal tone and a strong vagal brake. Schwartz (2018) suggests that "The tone of the vagus nerve is learned in early caregiver relationships. When those relationships aren't safe; the body doesn't feel safe". The process of co-regulation provides a platform from which attachment (Bowlby, 1988) can form and the infant can depend entirely on its caregiver through experiencing a felt sense of safety.

As therapists, we are often asked for help in supporting the client to develop self-regulation tools or strategies. The capacity for self-regulation is entirely dependent on whether co-regulation has first been experienced and whether the primary caregiver has offered safety and connection. Often, clients referred have not had the opportunity to practice self-soothing, because co-regulation has been lacking or limited during early development. Many have experienced misattunement or been left to try and desperately cope with nervous systems that have had no socially engaged influence.

Tom's nervous system was not developed in a safe environment. His first parent had a dysregulated nervous system and could not offer Tom the experience of co-regulation. In the playground, Tom was able to borrow his teacher's nervous system. Through the process of co-regulation, his teacher was able to move him from ALARM State to the AWAKE State. She offered him enough of a sense of safety so he could reduce his protective behaviours and move from the playground back into school. His nervous system trusted her nervous system. The teacher was able to intentionally influence Tom's protective position and bring him to a point where he was able to reengage in connection.

It is only through reciprocal regulation of our autonomic states that we feel safe to move into connection and create trusting relationships. This gives us a clear explanation as to why early healthy relationships encourage a psychological flexibility that supports the ability to overcome later challenges. Regardless of your therapeutic modality, the most important job a therapist has is to elicit a felt sense of safety so clients can build trust and move towards developing a sense of self. Lisa Dion describes how the therapist is the external regulator and how during the therapeutic process the child is "borrowing your nervous system" (2021) in the way that an infant would have sought to borrow their primary caregivers'. The therapeutic process is fundamentally, a neural exercise of the Social Engagement System. It offers our clients the opportunity to be in the AWAKE State alongside the presence of a caring, nurturing, and attuned adult.

With a foundational understanding of the neurobiological structure and process of the nervous system, we can start to conceptualise how clients present in the ANS 'A' States and consider the inevitable shifting between states that will take place during a session. Therapists have the privilege of being in the perfect position to intentionally influence their clients' nervous systems. By lending clients our nervous system and giving them the experience of co-regulation, we offer a neuroception of safety and the opportunity to develop a sense of self.

Chapter 4

Shaping Behaviour and Sense of Safety

There are a multitude of reasons why children come into our therapy rooms. Sometimes, it is a one-off event such as a bereavement which can cause caregivers to realise that within shared pain, they are unable to hold and manage their child's emotional process. More often, our caseload is filled with referrals for children who have had a difficult start in life. These clients are experiencing the long-term effects of growing up in an environment which did not meet their needs, causing them to develop in service of protection and survival.

Within this chapter, we will be exploring the various ways the behaviours seen in our clients are manifested and shaped. The nature/nurture debate has long been analysed and argued. The prevalent school of thought is that there is undoubtedly an intersection between the two. Whilst it is generally agreed that certain characteristics, for example, a vulnerability to some diseases or hair loss are inherited traits, emerging research shows that environmental factors such as traumatic events and trauma responses can change the way genes work and how the body reads a DNA sequence. Study into gene adaption is called epigenetics and it considers how environmental events essentially switch off or transform the way genes give instructions. For example, a malnourished child born to very tall parents may not grow to full height. On a cellular level, the human body forms and develops in the most dynamic way to survive. These adaptations strongly influence the development and trajectory of the brain, sensory-motor system and autonomic nervous system.

We will start by exploring Adverse Childhood Experiences (ACEs) as well as Attachment and Developmental Trauma through the lens of the Polyvagal Theory. These areas can have a critical impact on development and how the architecture of the nervous system is formed. Whilst these topics have been extensively written about and are undoubtedly familiar to you, we provide an opportunity to reconsider the impact of these interruptions on the regulatory capacity of the developing child. You will then be invited to consider your clients' presentation.

Autonomic States and levels of defence have a physiological presentation. Your client's facial muscles, breath, pupil dilation, tummy murmurings, and tone of

DOI: 10.4324/9781003412571-5

voice indicate their autonomic state and if they are experiencing a neuroception of safety or threat. Developing the ability to infer how open or closed to connection your client is, will be a crucial factor in case conceptualisation, goal setting, and next steps.

Whatever the circumstance for the referral, all clients will have experienced some level of adversity. It is important to note that not all adversity leads to trauma, which refers to a lasting emotional response to distressing, negative or intense event(s) that overwhelms a person's capacity to cope. Children can experience life-changing difficulties, without it becoming traumatic for them. Indeed, some of our referrals may have been made to prevent an event from becoming a trauma.

> *Hannah experienced parental separation in her formative years. Her parents made the decision that their marriage was no longer sustainable, and they would be happier living separately. Yet Hannah did not experience a traumatic reaction to this rupture in her environment.*

Resilience is a term that is often used to describe children who seem to cope with stress and change well. Yet there is a real danger in assuming that resilience is something you are born with; you either have it or you don't. In fact, resilience is an attribute that can only develop in children who have at least one relationship with a caregiver who is attuned, responsive and able to offer repair to relational ruptures that inevitably occur. In other words, those children who borrow their primary caregiver's nervous system and experience consistent co-regulation in times of stress develop high vagal tone, which supports them to regulate through the different states of activation when stressful events occur.

Adverse Childhood Experiences

When a client is referred, we meet with the primary caregiver to gather appropriate information on the needs and experiences of the child or young person. In effect, we are assessing the prevalence of ACEs for the primary caregiver and the client, which helps to inform case conceptualisation. Dr Vincent Felitti originally introduced the concept of ACEs in 1998. He was perplexed at the dropout rates of his patient's undergoing treatment for obesity. Dr Felitti found an anecdotal link between rates of obesity in adulthood and the experience of child sexual abuse. This led him to work alongside the Centres for Disease Control & Prevention to carry out a study to explore the association between childhood experiences and health throughout life. The original ACEs study (1998) involved 17,000 participants in the USA. It was the largest assessment of the association between negative experiences in childhood and health and well-being in adulthood.

ACEs are defined as being potentially traumatic events or situations that took place between the ages of 0 and 18, which may significantly affect a person's health and well-being. Felliti's ACEs study included three categories and asked adults for their experiences from the ages of 0 to 18 years:

- Abuse (physical, sexual, psychological)
- Neglect (physical, psychological)
- Family circumstances (domestic violence, substance abuse, parental separation or divorce, parental mental illness, parental incarceration).

The findings of the original study were eye-opening. They indicated a strong link between the prevalence of early adverse experiences and problematic outcomes in adulthood. Since the original study, countries and organisations across the globe have utilised the ACEs Questionnaire in an attempt to assess the needs of their communities and influence both local and global policy.

Research tells us that both physical and mental health can be impacted by ACEs. The more ACEs experienced appears to correlate with greater difficulties in adulthood. Data indicates a correlation between ACEs and an increase in the risk of cancer, heart disease, anxiety, depression, and PTSD. A Prisoner ACE survey conducted in Wales in 2018, found that individuals in the criminal justice system report higher levels of childhood adversity than those in the general population (Ford *et al.*, 2019).

It cannot be overstated how influential the ACEs study was in bringing attention to the relationship with adversity in childhood, health and well-being. There are concerns that the terms ACEs and Trauma are used interchangeably, without fully explaining why the experience of early adversity is more impactful for some children than others.

Reflecting on a changing society, any future ACE studies may need to expand the categories in the assessment. Alongside the inclusion of experiences of bereavement in childhood and bullying, we argue that living through COVID-19 is an ACE and should be included in future studies. The impact of living through the pandemic is only now being fully realised and will be explored at greater length in Chapter 9.

Case Conceptualisation is a key factor for therapists to understand and formulate potential treatment goals and ways of working with a client. An understanding of the impact of ACEs is important. However, they should not be considered as causal factors without having a good enough understanding of the child/young person's early history, including their relationships with primary caregivers. In addition, a curiosity about Positive Childhood Experiences (PCEs) is an important part of our intake process. Research indicates that PCEs and supportive relationships provide the shield that allows children to withstand, or recover, from adverse experiences (Sege *et al.*, 2017). From a polyvagal lens, we need to consider whether the nervous systems of our clients were soothed during any adversity experienced, or whether they were left in states of dysregulation.

Teddy was 2 years old when the global pandemic of COVID-19 arrived. He had to isolate with his grandparents who were deemed as vulnerable adults due to their ages and health difficulties. They were extremely frightened of contracting the disease. This period followed a developmentally harmful period wherein Teddy experienced at least five categorised ACEs (neglect, emotional abuse, domestic violence, parental drug use and parental incarceration). Throughout his early years, Teddy had multiple and consistent episodes of adversity without a responsive adult to support him to return to feelings of safety.

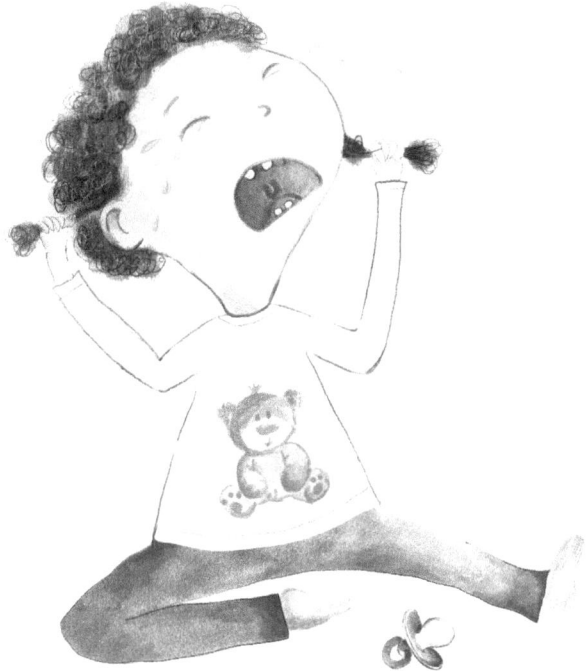

Figure 4.1 Teddy.

Human infants are altricial, which means that they arrive in the world underdeveloped, helpless, and dependent on parental care for an extended period. Ongoing and critical development of the brain, nervous system, motor system, and sensory system happens after birth and continues to do so. Whilst there continues to be raging debate about why the human design causes us to be the most underequipped of all mammals at birth, social psychology argues that 'being human' implies having the capacity for relationship, culture, language, and empathy. These need to be learned from our early caregivers. This is a highly risky evolutionary strategy, entirely dependent on the long-term commitment from caregivers to detect and respond to an infant's needs. Human caregivers need to have enough self-regulation to be optimally available to their infants whilst also experiencing necessary rupture and repair. Caregivers must provide shelter, warmth, and protection. They need to have the capacity to psychologically attune and soothe their infant's nervous system through the process of co-regulation.

Although infants and young children will inevitably move into hyper-aroused states of sympathetic activation, they are incapable of fighting, fleeing, or defending themselves in times of stress. Adults have an option to mobilise when they feel a sense of threat. Whereas babies and young children have evolved to attract the attention of their primary caregiver to protect and soothe their nervous system in situations of perceived danger. The demand for some primary caregivers to be a long-term external incubator for their infant to develop successfully is unattainable. For many babies and children, the adult who should offer protection may instead be the source of fear or perpetrator of neglect. The resultant outcome is Developmental Trauma which has been referred to by van der Kolk (2009) and Busuttil (2009) as "exposure to multiple, cumulative traumatic events, usually of an interpersonal nature, during childhood which results in developmentally adverse consequences". Put another way, developmental trauma typically occurs through repeated traumatic experiences of abuse, neglect, or unmet attachment needs. It most often happens in the carer/child dyad during the early years and/or at times of significant development, including in utero.

Developmental Trauma

Often referred to as Childhood Trauma or Early Trauma, we feel that 'Developmental' is a highly relevant descriptor as it reminds us that repeated and pervasive negative experiences occur during the most critical period in the human lifespan. The human brain starts its 20-plus-year journey of maturation at approximately 2 weeks after conception (Tierney & Nelson, 2009) and is heavily influenced by environmental factors. Whilst brain development continues into the early-20s, the most environmentally impactful time for the formation of a healthy brain is during the early childhood years where foundations are laid. This provides the neural platform so that higher brain regions can grow and be accessible later in life.

As with the development of the ANS, the brain develops in a hierarchical manner. Starting with the functions necessary for immediate survival (respiration) and finishing with brain areas that are most complex and dispensable, influencing behaviour and thought. During foetal development, neurons are created and migrate to form the various brain regions. Whilst the basic architecture of the brain is formed before birth, neural complexity and growth occurs long afterwards and is dependent on the care received.

Sitting just above the spinal cord, the first brain region to develop is the brain stem, from which the vagus nerve emerges. Almost fully developed by the second trimester, the brain stem houses sensory pathways and, is responsible for the internal survival system (breathing, temperature, heart rate, impulses) and instinctual fight-flight reactions to threat. Figure 4.2 illustrates three regions of the brain.

The limbic system develops next and plays a crucial role in how we respond to stressful situations and is strongly associated with attachment functions (Schore, 2001). Achieving a high level of maturity by 8 months gestation (Cozolino, 2006) this brain region supports the evaluation of danger and works to mediate the primal fight-flight instincts, acting like an emotion-processing centre

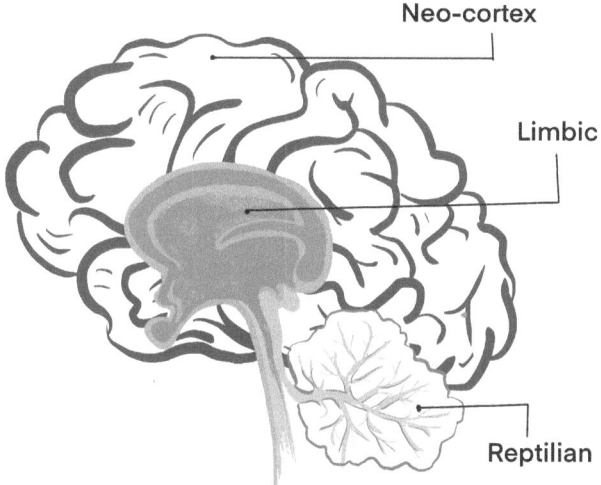

Neo-cortex

Limbic

Reptilian

Figure 4.2 Brain regions.

(Schore, 2001). If threat signals are perceived, the amygdala alerts the hypothalamus which activates the sympathetic nervous system, generating the hormone epinephrine (also known as adrenaline), and moves our body into the ALARM State.

The cortex is the final area of the brain to develop. Full maturation of this brain region is not complete until early adulthood, giving a much longer window for developmental disruption to occur (Murphy et al., 2022). Access to this region of the brain is only fully attainable when we are in the AWAKE State, and we are vagally mediated.

As the nervous system develops and grows, it can start to organise and influence our more primitive instinctual responses. A newborn baby needs only to be able to breathe, cry, digest, and have a beating heart. As an altricial experience-dependent species, there is no evolutionary requirement for the use of language or abstract thought. However, by the age of 6 years, the influence of the limbic-cortical region on the instinctual brain stem is needed to enable learning, socialisation, and play. Concurrently, the development of vagal tone will influence the child's capacity to move into stressful situations without tipping into the ALARM State. As we grow, our brains need to become more complex to help us become more independent, learn skills, have a sense of self and form relationships. The capacity for higher brain regions to control the reactive lower brain regions is highly dependent on early experiences, and how effectively the ANS was soothed and supported to return to the AWAKE state in times of dysregulation.

As we have discussed, the human infant is born ready to be intentionally influenced by the care it receives and the environment it is born into. The term neural plasticity is used to describe the incredible changes the nervous system makes in response to its environment. The pervasive impact developmental trauma has on the structural organisation and functional capabilities of the brain has been demonstrated (Perry, 1999, p. 2006; Schore, 2000, 2001). If an immature nervous system grows in an environment enveloped in toxic stress, the nervous system will develop in ways to survive and adapt to this environment. Through his extensive research on the impact of trauma on the brain, Dr Bruce Perry, an expert in brain development and childhood trauma, explains how during early brain development there are critical, sensitive periods of neural organisation which require specific organising experiences (1999). If those experiences are missed or disrupted due to either lack of either sensory experience or extremes of experience, deficits in neurodevelopment can be seen. To illustrate this, he invites us to consider how not being touched for 2 weeks could have devastating effects on a baby, whilst a 12-year-old child may be able to tolerate this. The baby needs to be touched in a loving, caring, sensitive way to grow, and feel safe and secure. Primarily it will communicate its needs through its body and social engagement system. If those needs are not met, the baby will adapt and change, finding the best way to keep their primary caregiver close to them. These adaptations are referred to as Attachment Strategies. We argue that all attachment strategies should be looked upon as strengths. Behaviours are shaped and modified in service of survival.

Tom, Teddy, and Emma have all experienced Developmental Trauma. Whilst their symptoms are expressed very differently, all have adapted individual strategies to survive the environments into which they were born. They all experience relational difficulties within their families and amongst their peer group. Their adversities took place during sensitive periods of neural organisation resulting in low vagal tone, primed to protect rather than connect. Their experiences have affected their capacity to access higher brain regions. Although none have a diagnosis, they are all finding it challenging to learn requiring additional support in the classroom/nursery.

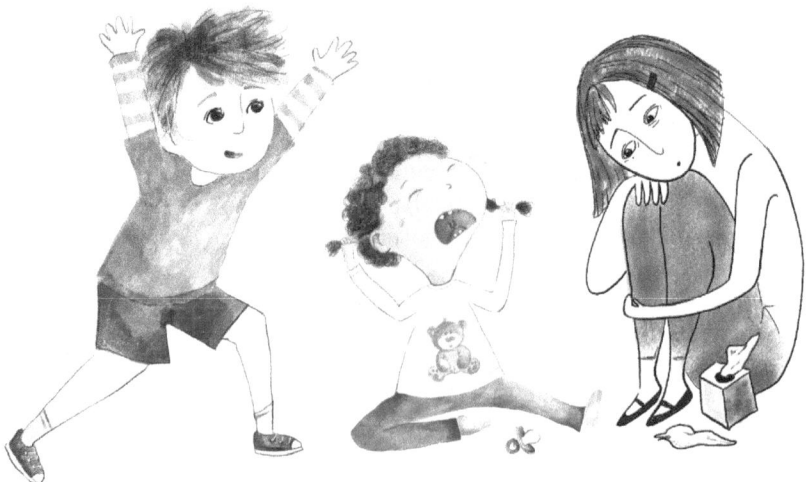

Figure 4.3 Tom, Teddy, and Emma.

Attachment

With the development of neuroscience, it is now proffered that John Bowlby's attachment theory is a theory of regulation (Schore, 2000). Bowlby sought to answer the question as to why early interpersonal relationships between an infant and their primary caregiver impacted on the human life experience. The basic premise of Bowlby's ground-breaking theory is that to survive, the infant will seek proximity to their primary caregiver (primary attachment figure) and will become distressed when their primary caregiver is not close by. Through a reciprocal relationship the primary caregiver will become attuned to the cues of the infant and respond consistently, creating a safe base from which the infant can develop a sense of safety (internal working model) forming the foundation for healthy identity development.

Bowlby built his theory from a multi-disciplinary lens drawing from evolutionary biology, developmental psychology, psychoanalysis, cognitive science, and ethology. From the earliest days he insisted that to begin to understand this complex and unique interpersonal system, one must explore it from all scientific angles. Modern attachment theorists have built upon Bowlby's theory through the inclusion of wider disciplines, including but not limited to: Anthropology, Developmental Psychopathology, Clinical Psychology, Mentalisation, Linguistics, Neuroscience, Neuropsychology, Mathematics, Physics, and Sociology. All come to the same fundamental conclusion that attachment is the dyadic regulation of emotion.

Allan Schore explains that "Bowlby's original descriptions occurred during a period of behaviorism" (2007). Through advances in neuroscience and neuropsychology we now understand that whilst Bowlby's theory remains highly relevant, attachment is not a behavioural process but rather a bodily based process. Psychobiological attunement and the quality of the relationship in the infant-carer dyad impacts on the development of the brain and nervous system as a result of neural plasticity and epigenetics. Schore (1994) offers that the quality of attachment has a critical influence on the development of the right brain system which is involved in "processing of emotion, modulation of stress, self-regulation, and thereby the functional origins of the bodily-based implicit self". We therefore understand that the development of attachment is far more consequential than behavioural outcomes resulting from the experience of feeling safe and secure.

There is a plethora of scientific research which proves that the attachment process impacts on physiological development. Through his development on Reflective Functioning (Fonagy *et al.*, 1991), Fonagy provides us with a 'how' of attachment theory. Reflective functioning is the action a person takes as a result of their capacity to understand the mental states of another whilst processing their own internal states. An attuned primary caregiver understands that their infant has thoughts, feelings, emotions, and experiences that are different from their own. In turn, they make links for the infant by interpreting their mental and resultant behaviour. Reflective functioning is considered a crucial aspect in the development of an infant's regulatory capacity. Furthermore, the Polyvagal Theory explains how the attachment process supports the development of high vagal tone, and the capacity to return to social engagement through the repeated experiences of the consistent co-regulation of the caregiver during the first 3 years of life.

A standard intake meeting for new clients includes a discussion with the primary caregiver about the child's birth and early years' experience. Claire beamed with joy when sharing her memories of Hannah's earliest moments. "We were a team! She seemed to be able to tell me what she needed from the beginning. If I didn't know, I asked her, even though I knew she couldn't understand me! Hannah loved me singing to her. If she cried, I used to dance around the kitchen with her". Claire was containing and mirroring Hannah's energy, co-regulating with her child. She was able to understand that baby Hannah was having her own thoughts and feelings. Claire used song, touch, and prosody to attune to Hannah's needs, soothing her nervous system and supporting the development of attachment security.

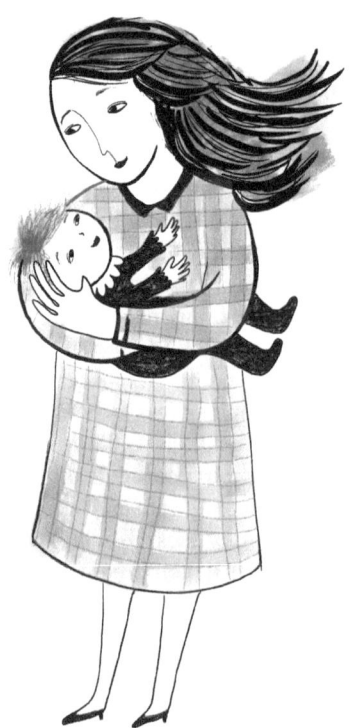

Figure 4.4 Hannah and Claire.

A child's earliest attachment involves numerous experiences of rupture and repair where the child moves between states of autonomic dysregulation and regulation (Hadiprodjo, 2018).

For the primary caregiver to mentalise, be reflective and offer co-regulation, their nervous system must be vagally mediated. The primary caregiver will be in the AWAKE State and have the capacity to create a 'holding environment' (Winnicott, 1953) for their baby. This influences the development of the vagal brake and the eventual maturation of self-regulation.

When a primary caregiver soothes their baby, they are essentially soothing the baby's nervous system. A baby who does not experience having their nervous system soothed in times of stress, does not learn how to adequately regulate their emotions.

Amira is an infant who communicates her distress through her body. It has been observed that Layla and Ali handle Amira very roughly, are not attentive, responsive, or sensitive to her needs. In the presence of Layla, Amira smiles and tries to catch her mum's 'eye'. Amira is more animated with Layla and often moves her body and has more dribble in her mouth. Amira is in the ALARM State. In the presence of Ali, Amira either arches her back or goes floppy. This is dependent on how Ali uses his body and the loudness of his voice. When Ali is intrusive or picking Amira up in a rough manner, she turns her head and avoids eye contact. Amira does not attempt to engage with Ali. Amira is in the AVOID State. We see that neither Layla or Ali are mentalising or co-regulating. Amira's autonomic nervous system is not being soothed. She experiences frequent attachment ruptures without repair.

Many of the children who come into our therapy rooms have not had the experience of a soothed nervous system. Therapy must act on the stress response systems of the brain and nervous system and regulate a child's arousal if it is to be effective (Schore, 2001; Levine & Kline, 2006). In so doing, therapists can provide a developmentally corrective experience of attachment for those children who have missed out on this early experience. The therapist can serve as a secondary attachment figure through lending the client their nervous system.

Take a moment to consider the primary reasons your current clients have been referred to you for therapeutic support. It is possible that you have been asked to support children presenting with one of the following difficulties:

- Concentration difficulties
- Oppositional behaviours
- Anger Management
- Experience of domestic violence
- Processing parental separation
- Hyperactivity

- Relating to peers
- Processing grief and/or loss
- Developmental trauma
- Withdrawn behaviour

Reframing these presenting issues through the lens of the Polyvagal Theory, we consider that the above concerns are challenges with self-regulation. In an interview for the Psychotherapy Networker, Dr Daniel Siegel stated, "Almost every mental health problem; anxiety, depression, eating disorders, personality disorders, thinking disorders are issues of self-regulation" (2012). Whether you refer to the work of Allan Schore (1994, 2001), Dan Siegel and Tina Payne Bryson (2011), Lisa Dion (2018), or Gabor Maté and Daniel Maté (2022), all are curious about emotion regulation. Their work seeks to explain and explore how the body's regulatory capacity is formed. How it informs future relationships, perceptions of the world and the capacity to engage in society at large.

Our Six Storytellers have self-regulation challenges. Teddy, Tom, Amira and Emma have mismatched nervous systems arising from developmental trauma and adverse early experiences. They have low vagal tone and struggle to experience prolonged neuroception of safety. Hannah has both experienced significant loss and disruption due to the death of an important secondary attachment figures during the COVID 19 pandemic. Ezra experienced a body trauma when he was an infant. He has a reduced vagal tone due to his burn injury and infections that he has been treated for post-surgeries. It is also possible that he has vagus nerve dysfunction because of physical and psychological stress recently compounded by COVID-19 and his parents current relationship difficulties.

Identifying a Mismatched Smoke Alarm

The physiological connection between facial/neck/ear muscles and the beating heart demonstrates expressions and tone of voice used to communicate the state of our ANS. A smiling face and rhythmic voice tell another: "I have a steady heartbeat, I am not frightened or frightening, I want to connect with you". A flat, expressionless face says: "I am defensive. My heartbeat is unsteady. I am not feeling safe, I am not able to connect with you".

It is almost impossible to maintain face-to-face gaze or focus on the sound of another person speaking when your heart is racing, and you are in the ALARM State. The muscles around the mouth are not moved to smile. You cannot speak in a melodic way when your heart rate is decreased, and you are in the AVOID State. When children are in the AWAKE State, they are expressive and receptive with a strong face-to-heart connection. They have natural vocal intonation, speak with rhythm, smile, and play. Figure 4.5 illustrates the face-to-heart connection.

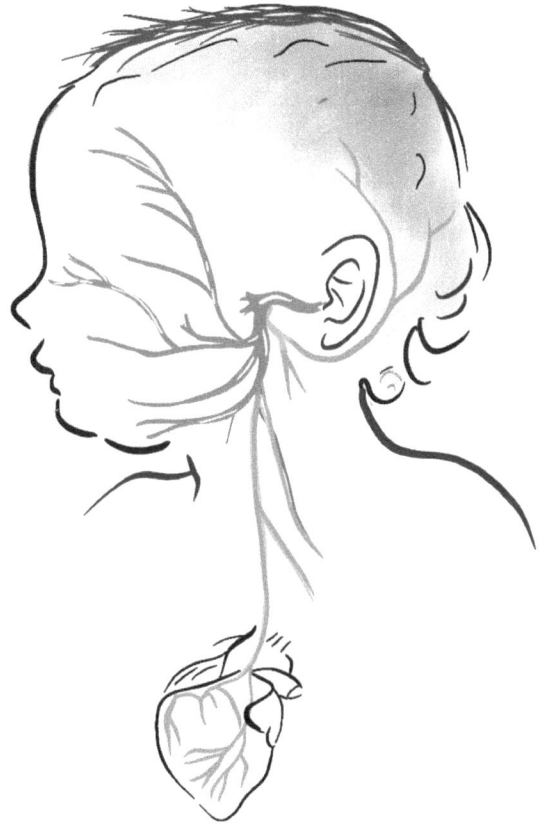

Figure 4.5 Face-to-heart connection.

From the moment we first meet a client, they will be offering us plenty of nonverbal clues which communicate whether they have a felt sense of safety or are in a defensive state. Clients with sensitive smoke alarm will present their protective positions through physiological markers. Paying attention to these, therapists become aware of potential dysregulation and autonomic shifts. The following questions invite inquiry into the client's physiological presentation:

Physiological Aspect	Curiosity Questions
Voice	Does your client speak rhythmically? Is the volume and tone of their voice in context with what they are saying or doing? Do they have any speech difficulties?
Sound	Is the client highly responsive to even the smallest of sounds? Do they respond to your voice? Can they hear what you are saying? Can your client follow your instructions? Can they retain information?
Facial expressions	What is your client's face telling you? Do they have flat, expressionless faces? Is there spontaneity in the upper part of their face? Do their eyes crinkle when they smile? Do their expressions feel too much and not in keeping with their story or game?
Eye Gaze	Is your client able to look you in the eye and offer face-to-face gaze? Are their pupils dilated or like pinpricks? Does it seem like they have no peripheral vision, and they are staring in one place?
Gut and Bowel	Does your client suddenly need to go the toilet? Are they farting or burping? Is their tummy making lots of sounds and gurgling noises?

We may describe clients as either hyper-aroused or hypo-aroused. Through a polyvagal lens we can consider how that these energetic positions come from an involuntary reaction with bodies stuck in a trauma response mode. As you consider these physiological markers, you are beginning to formulate an understanding of your client's vagal tone. Feeling safe does not happen just because there is no threat in the here and now. A child with high vagal tone will respond playfully to a therapeutic space that is safe and welcoming. In contrast to a child with a low vagal tone who presents with a lack of prosody, poor face-to-face gaze, incongruent facial expressivity, and a sensitivity to sound. Their Super Protector© is unable to distinguish a real threat from a perceived threat, they have a faulty smoke alarm.

During early therapy sessions, Emma presented with flat affect. She avoided eye contact and had no rhythm to her voice. Her body movements were very slow and heavy, she would stand at the edge of the room unable to decide where to sit or what to do. Emma was unable to distinguish whether she was hot or cold, thirsty, or hungry. In the therapy room she would engage with the sandtray often creating scenes with the animal miniatures. She rarely made accompanying sounds or noises when interacting with the toys. Physiological markers demonstrated that Emma's neural circuits were unable to distinguish whether situations or people were safe or dangerous, causing an inability to inhibit her defence systems in a safe environment.

If a child's ANS has developed during the conditions we described earlier, they will have a highly reactive Smoke Alarm system. The evolutionary imperative to

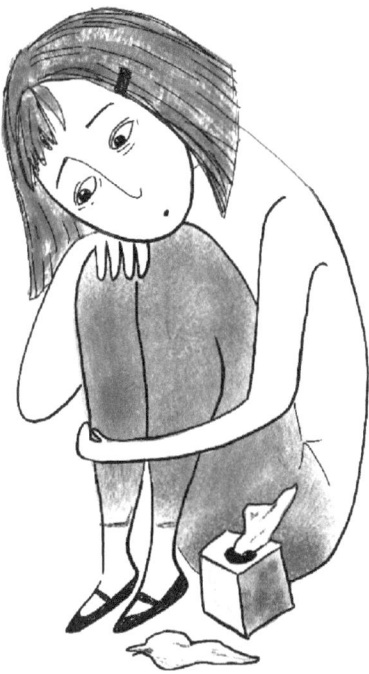

Figure 4.6 Emma.

seek connection with others will have been replaced by a protective stance. From this position, seeking connection is not experienced as safe and is not in service of survival. Instead, their ANS has developed a habitual defensive response resulting in distorted social awareness. The adaptive seeking of social connection becomes replaced, the client is transported to their accustomed position of either ALARM or AVOID.

> *Ezra finds the classroom environment overwhelming. He cannot move around easily and uses walking sticks. He can present as angry and has been known to throw his walking sticks when in the classroom. He is in the ALARM State. The teacher evacuates the classroom and Ezra is left on his own. Nobody will enter the classroom until they see that Ezra has 'calmed down'. He then moves into the AVOID State. We see that Ezra has a highly reactive Smoke Alarm as he protects himself within the school environment moving between sympathetic and dorsal vagal.*

As therapists, we often find that children with a mismatched smoke alarm find transitions and change particularly challenging. Porges describes how mammalian animals thrive on novelty if it is experienced in a safe environment. Small children will rush off to play at a new soft play centre; puppies will move from their mother to rough and tumble together; kittens will explore new heights and jump

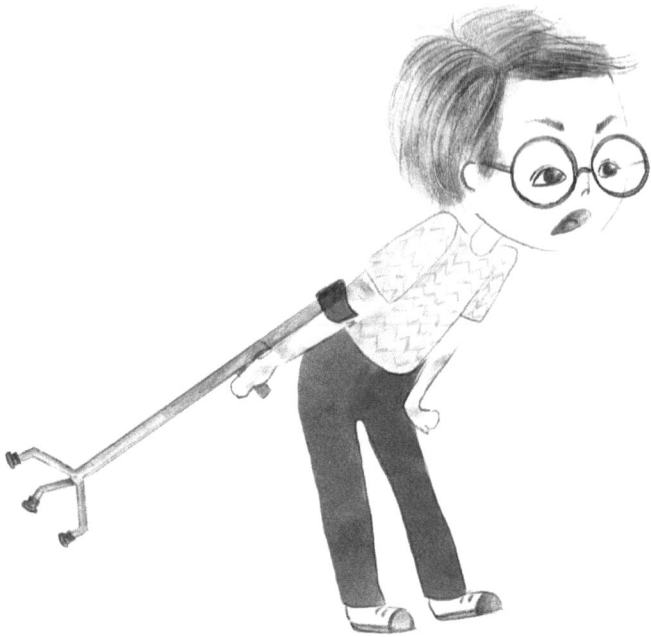

Figure 4.7 Ezra.

on curtains. In all cases, this exploration and curiosity can take place because they have the physiological blueprint which tells them that they can return to mother if frightened, and experience co-regulation leading to a safe and social position. Children who are traumatised do not have that path to safety and will not risk novel experiences.

Antonio Damasio (2003) tells us that, "emotions are played out in the theatre of the body". We know that these protective stances are involuntary. These happen to our clients which means that their fear isn't consciously known either. Oftentimes they will be experiencing and communicating protective emotions on a bodily level without even knowing they are feeling these feelings.

Children in the ALARM State have a very active relationship with the environment. They are hyperalert to environmental changes and have high levels of energy and are primed in any of the following ways:

- sound sensitivity is elevated
- eye muscles allow more light with improved far vision
- heart rate increases
- adrenaline is activated.

Children in the AVOID State have ended their relationship with the environment. They have shut down their feelings to conserve energy and protect themselves from pain as well as:

- being closed off to environmental factors
- having constricted pupils
- experiencing deadened sound

Tracking a client's presentation will help therapists consider if a client can move between states according to matched or mismatched neuroception. A client who is in the AWAKE State is open to connection with you. A client who is in the ALARM State or AVOID State will be rigidly protective.

We have developed a brief checklist, the Physiological Markers Checklist: PMC© to help you consider how your clients present and use as part of your Case Conceptualisation. This tool encourages therapists to have focused awareness of clients' unconscious non-verbal communication about their internal worlds. When utilised throughout the therapeutic process, it serves as an additional measure of the client's development of a neuroception of safety.

This checklist is intended to be used as a component in the case conceptualisation process. Whilst it utilises a scoring system, we acknowledge that the PMC is subjective and does not in and of itself identify vagal function or consider any variabilities arising from a diagnosis. The PMC can be applied to your work with children aged 4 years old to 16 years old. Cultural considerations always need to be held. Its main purpose is to offer a baseline from which the therapist can consider whether it is necessary to focus on procuring a sense of safety for the client (Figure 4.8).

The PMC is divided into five physiological categories: Vocal, Auditory, Facial Expression, Eye Gaze, and Gut and Bowel. Each relate to external markers that indicate whether a child or young person feels safe or is responding to a perceived threat. Each statement within these categories is scored from 0 to 4, and the total score is the sum of all five category scores, with a maximum possible score of 68, indicating a high perception of threat. The PMC is available to download for free at www.pipsolutions.co.uk, with full details on scoring. It must be emphasised that the PMC is not a diagnostic tool but is intended to aid case conceptualisation through a polyvagal perspective.

The PMC can help us consider whether the novelty of the therapeutic space may be overwhelming for some clients. It is highly likely for children who did not have core conditions met by an early caregiver will have a mismatched nervous system. They may respond with involuntary protective behaviours which need to be attended to and held before therapeutic intervention is applied.

PMC   ### Physiological Markers Checklist©

The PMC is a brief assessment tool which helps you consider your client's autonomic activation in the therapy room. The PMC is designed as a component in the case conceptualisation process and does not in and of itself identify vagal function. Below are statements describing physiological markers.

For each statement, tick the box which best describes your client:

0 – Never / 1 – Rarely / 2 Occasionally / 3 Frequently / 4 Always

	0	1	2	3	4
Vocal					
Speaks in a monotone voice					
Speaks with inappropriate volume					
Vocal Score					
Auditory					
Unresponsive to your voice					
Unable to follow instructions					
Unable to read or respond your vocal prosody					
Reactive to ambient noise					
Auditory Score					
Facial Expression					
Lack of spontaneity in the upper part of their face					
Eyes don't crinkle when smiling					
Flat facial affect					
Facial Expression Score					
Eye Gaze					
Unable to sustain eye contact					
Unable to offer face to face gaze					
Dilated pupils					
Constricted pupils					
Fixed gaze					
Eye Gaze Score					
Gut and Bowel					
Makes frequent visits to toilet					
Release of gas (farting/burping)					
Digestion sounds/tummy gurgling					
Gut and Bowel Score					
Total Score					

Physiological Markers Checklist©: PMC 2024 O'Neill & McDonald   Free to download @ www.pipsolutions.co.uk

Figure 4.8 Physiological Markers Checklist: PMC ©.

The Needs Paradox®

The healthy development of Attachment Security, Neurobiological functioning, Emotion Regulation, Sensory Motor Processing and Vagal Tone all rely on a set of conditions being met during specific developmental windows. All these processes are integrated and flourish through the experience of a co-regulated, holding environment wherein the primary caregiver interprets, contains, mirrors, and offers an attuned response to their infant's myriad communications of happiness, stress, frustration, and fear. Children who have had co-regulation withdrawn or offered inconsistently, unconsciously learn not to trust the potential of relying on a safe adult. Their nervous system will not have had exposure to a ventral vagally mediated nervous system. Co-regulation, the very thing that is needed to support the development of a high Vagal Tone and a functioning Vagal Brake, is perceived as dangerous to a nervous system enveloped by trauma. We define this dilemma as "The Needs Paradox®".

> *Emma was fully entrenched in The Needs Paradox®. From her time in the womb, she experienced life-threatening violence, domestic instability. Furthermore, she is currently living in a household where physical aggression is an ongoing threat. Emma developed incredible strategies to ensure survival. She learnt that relationships with adults are dangerous, recruiting an almost persistent AVOID State, feeling nothing at all to mitigate pain and suffering. To develop high vagal tone and be able to access her social engagement system, Emma needed to experience repeated offerings of attunement and co-regulation. A neuroception of safety was necessary before she could contemplate a reciprocal relationship with an adult.*

Children living within a dysregulated body have had repeated, ongoing ruptures without receiving the opportunity to repair. The way a child or young person communicates is related to the emotional feedback originated in the primary caregiver-infant dyad. If there is minimal repair, the unconscious belief will be that the rupture is more important.

As therapists, we understand that healing can only manifest within the repeated experience of co-regulation, attunement and empathy. Ruptures are a necessary component in the therapeutic process and provide us with golden moments wherein we can offer a new experience for our clients, increasing the potential for lasting change. Offering a 're-do' of these conditions is the basis of positive therapeutic intervention. Yet, what our clients need to heal can be perceived as terrifying: The Needs Paradox®. There will be inevitable moments when our attempts to offer these core conditions to our clients will trigger their habituated active ALARM State or hidden AVOID State. This is not disastrous.

Until your client has repeated experiences of cues of safety from you, their nervous systems will be unable to contemplate that the therapeutic process might not be threatening to them. Adverse events themselves do not result in pervasive damage, rather it is when ruptures and injuries occur in the absence of a protective relationship trauma is established.

As a therapist you are offering to take the role of the good enough therapist, wherein you will provide your clients repeated, positive experiences leading to lasting change. Through eliciting a neuroception of safety you are able to intentionally impact the neurobiology of your clients. By repairing a rupture, the therapist is modelling how to withstand shame and offers the potential of a different relationship.

Studies into epigenetics, including 'Early Experiences Can Alter Gene Expression and Affect Long-Term Development' (2010), tell us that changes to the way genes process information are reversible. Neural plasticity enables the nervous system to reorganise itself by forming new neural connections. Through the lens of the Polyvagal Theory, we come to understand that in borrowing your nervous system clients are supported to move from patterns of protection to patterns of connection, eventually developing high vagal tone. As therapists, whether intentionally or not, our own autonomic states will impact our clients and vice versa. It is therefore imperative that we have an awareness of our own states, triggers, and window of tolerance. In the next chapter we will introduce you to your own nervous system and the concept of the therapist as the Emotional Regulator.

Chapter 5

Emotional Regulator

In the previous chapter, we considered how regardless of the reason for a referral, children who come to therapy for support are likely to be struggling to self-regulate in the face of adversity and stress. The therapeutic process can effect real change within a child's neurobiology, especially in re-balancing the physiology of the stress response system. This will happen if the therapist is able to communicate cues of safety and a steady stream of play signals, keeping the child within their autonomic window of tolerance. In so doing, the therapist is relationally regulating their client's nervous system, ultimately leading to the development of self-regulation.

Often a referrer's main target for their child's therapy is self-regulation. Through the lens of the Polyvagal Theory, we understand that without the ability to move through different states of activation and return to a desire for connection, the world is very lonely, frightening, and confusing. A lack of self-regulation in children is the cause of many challenging behaviours which create difficulties for adults, whether they are trying to parent or teach.

Through the process of neuroception, our nervous system is constantly scanning for cues of safety or threat and will be moving through various autonomic states throughout the day. Those of us with high vagal tone will be able to move between the bidirectional ANS 'A' States: AWAKE, ALARM, AVOID, often without even realising it has happened. When facing stress, a strong vagal brake enables us to seek connection, and the world is experienced as fundamentally safe. Utilising our social engagement system, we bypass the need to protect ourselves. Regulation does not mean we are always calm. Rather, it refers to the capacity to return to a position of 'okayness', following moment-by-moment environmental, relational, and internal triggers that have been responded to with appropriate energy.

There are beliefs that therapists should be able to hold each session through a vagally mediated nervous system. Whatever our clients do or say, we should remain in the AWAKE State, regulated and containing. Our emotional world should be ignored with an exclusive focus on the needs and affect changes in our clients. Yet we now know that this isn't humanly possible. Our nervous system is designed to move through adaptive states in response to the data it is presented with, sometimes we will be triggered. Our nervous system does not switch off because we have our therapist hat on and nor should it.

DOI: 10.4324/9781003412571-6

Children do not have the capacity to effectively utilise full cortical functioning. They will be processing and responding from a sensorimotor, bottom-up, right-brain, limbic system. They will more often express their difficulties and trauma experiences through their body rather than their words. It is therefore essential that we can utilise the non-verbal, somatic information our body is receiving from our clients. An attuned therapist will be mindful to the feelings and changes in their own body, in response to their client's unconscious communications. Schore (2015) describes how the feelings are experienced in the therapist as "subjective interoceptive autonomic responses". In other words, therapists will themselves experience a shared embodied experience with their clients whether they like it or not!

Within this chapter, we will explore the interpersonal processes of Transference and Countertransference. As an endemic component within the therapeutic dyad, these processes provide us with rich detail that can be used to support the client in developing healthier relational interactions. Alternatively, each of these mental mechanisms has the potential to precipitate difficult feelings in the therapist, causing autonomic protective responses to emerge. Linking such concepts to a Polyvagal framework can help us organise ourselves, remove any self-judgement and enable a re-establishment of connection, allowing us to offer our clients a sense that relationships are repairable and co-regulation is safe.

Sometimes we will have an explicit awareness that the non-verbal communication, behaviour, story or play offered to us by our clients is causing us to have big feelings both sensorily and emotionally. However, if we haven't explored our own triggers and autonomic states, we will move into involuntary protection without any awareness. Our ANS will have gone to work valiantly, performing as it is designed to. Therapeutic work with children is rarely a cognitive process. An attuned therapist can never simply be a witness to their client's experience. They will always join the journey and feel their client's feelings, whilst working to remain intersubjective.

Being truly familiar with our autonomic states could be considered an ethical imperative. Schore and Schore (2007) describe the psychobiological core to the therapeutic relationship, where the therapist serves as an attuned nervous system regulator. If we are blind to our triggers and protective positions, we will be unable to offer attunement and instead may be attempting to lend a dysregulated system to the children in our care. To do our work effectively and look after ourselves in the process, we must get to know our own nervous systems. Lisa Dion (2018) considers that the fundamental cause of therapist burnout is the unattended dysregulation of their own nervous systems, and we wholeheartedly agree. Our nervous system will become entangled with those of our clients, working hard to return to ventral activation and transmit cues of safety whilst simultaneously seeking and translating our clients' non-verbal signals. The repeated offering up of ourselves to children who bring with them a system built to protect itself is exhausting and the need to attend to our own wellbeing cannot be overemphasised.

Through a variety of activities and exercises, this chapter will introduce you to your own Autonomic Nervous System. You are invited to be curious about your personal experience of each autonomic state. The activities offered will help you bring to conscious awareness which position your nervous system is most familiar with in times of stress. We will also consider what circumstances might bring you there. Finally, we will think about how you can move back to connection and integrate this process in your therapy sessions.

Who Are You a Container for?

The role of a child therapist invites many opportunities to practice self-regulation! Our job requires us to be relationally involved with people bringing their worries and difficult experiences for us to hear and hold. Teachers, parents, grandparents, foster-carers, social workers, children are all invested in our ability to facilitate change. Therapists who work with children often find they have multiple relationships attached to one client.

As we have learned, the Polyvagal Theory's position explains how, providing we have access to the ventral vagal position, we can offer co-regulation and support a reduction in the physiological stress response system. It would be naïve to think that this is the only process at play in the therapy room. This non-verbal exchange happens in tandem with the bidirectional communication between the mind of the person we are working with, within which the mental mechanisms of transference and countertransference will be oscillating, resulting in thoughts, feelings and emotions shared by the therapist and the client.

Transference

In her first meeting with Tom's parents, the therapist became quickly alert to a level of tension and anxiety in Michelle, Tom's mother. They were 2 minutes late for the meeting, for which she apologised profusely. In response to the therapist's offer of a hot drink she replied, "there's no need to go to any trouble for us". During the meeting, Michelle seemed to play down her husband's description of Tom's behaviour, insisting that he is a lovely boy, and they are the luckiest parents in the world. When the therapist gently enquired about their experience of parenting Tom, Michelle was insistent that whilst it was sometimes tricky, they wouldn't change a thing. She commented, "he is probably just going through a wobbly stage". Michelle described how she has read all the books recommended to her by social workers and school, emphasising her gratitude that the therapist would be supporting their family.

In subsequent meetings, Michelle shared that her only dream was to be a mother. As adoptive parents, Michelle and Paul will have been required to interact with multiple professionals to finally have their longed-for child. Michelle's perception was that professionals were only involved in her life to assess and judge her suitability to parent. She was permanently afraid that Tom would be removed if she wasn't good enough. Michelle perceived all professionals as threatening. Transferentially and unconsciously, she was positioning the therapist as another professional who may take her child away.

Transference is ubiquitous and as a child therapist we are involved in many professional relationships. The moment we interact with another human we bring our history. Our present is unconsciously experienced through the lens of our past and the past is often acted out in the present. This applies to everybody. All human interactions are be guided by internal representations of people and relationships shaped by their past experiences.

Bowlby introduced us to the concept of the Internal Working Model. This relational template and representation of parents laid down in neural networks are formed during infancy. In the context of transference, clients and caregivers unconsciously respond to us "as if" we are another from their past. Coupled with mismatched neuroception, many people we support will have a nervous system primed to perceive us as threatening. That is not to say that we are never experienced as safe. The therapist's position as new person in the life of their client, results in them unconsciously seeking ways to make sense of who we are and how we might relate to them. All our clients know are the experiences that they have had.

For many of our clients, the invitation to have a relationship with an attuned and curious adult is new. The Needs Paradox® explored in earlier chapters shows that warmth and empathy offered may be perceived as untrustworthy, triggering our clients to their habituated active ALARM State or hidden AVOID State. As therapists (or other professionals) this may place us in multiple representational positions:

- Kindness and sharing of the creative toolkit may position us as the *perfect parent*
- Limits and boundaries could evoke the *abusive parent*
- On ending the session, we may become the *rejecting parent*
- Providing consistency and safety we might be experienced as a *saviour*
- A glimpse of another client in the waiting room might illicit the *abandoner*
- Winning a game may occupy the role of the *bully*

Betty and Charles report that staff at the nursery where Teddy attends are kind and caring. Betty reported that they have a 'soft spot' for him as there is "something very endearing and charming about him". Betty has witnessed them being warm, nurturing, and empathic. Teddy may perceive moments of empathy and warmth from staff as untrustworthy triggering an ACTIVE Alarm State. Within Teddy's experiences and according to the framework of The Needs Paradox®, it can be hypothesised that the representational positions taken by staff are abusive parent, rejecting parent and abandoner. Teddy's behaviour shows that in the presence of caring nursery staff his original psychobiological wound from his early life experiences with Jemma is fully opened in the here and now. During his play therapy sessions, the therapist will apply the framework of The Needs Paradox® including co-regulation, attunement and therapeutic care.

Transference has long been considered a useful medium through which therapists can afford change for their clients. However, this can only happen if the therapist is consciously aware of the transference and is able to self-regulate through any difficult thoughts or feelings they have in response. If the therapist is left in the unconscious realm and their ANS is activated, client actions and affect may become impactful and countertransference will emerge.

Countertransference

Countertransference is commonly understood to be the therapists' response to a client's transference resulting in feelings, thoughts, images and/or dreams experienced by the therapist in relation to their client.

Whilst it is not mandatory, we would assume that practitioners working with children have afforded the time and space to have their personal own therapy. How therapists think and feel about themselves and others is no different to other humans. We are shaped and influenced by early experiences, attachment figures and how effectively our ANS was regulated. We were all children who have experienced disappointment, loss, shame, ruptures, repairs, wishes and dreams. Our earliest experiences were formed and held subcortically. An invitation to join our clients' non-verbal worlds can evoke powerful feelings and wake up implicit memories without warning. It is important to remember that working therapeutically with dysregulated children can be triggering.

Cozolino (2004) notes that the therapy room is a crowded place. The client brings with them their family, teachers, siblings and other key relationships. The therapist does the same. The professional 'choices' we have made will be influenced by our early history, family dynamics and desire to be a caretaker. Deciding to become a child and/or adolescent therapist, having a favoured client age range, studying a specific therapeutic modality and working in a particular environment, is unconsciously motivated by our personal history.

Countertransference never declares itself. It creeps in and responds to the behaviours and presentation of our clients. This can be conceptualised as transference in reverse. The unconscious influence that a therapist's past needs have on professional relationships.

Thinking about Hannah who was grieving for her grandmother. In therapy sessions the therapist observed Hannah's ability to self-regulate and her capacity to utilise more cognitive strategies to support herself. Hannah had good enough internal and external resources, with a neural expectation of safety. The therapist looked forward to seeing Hannah, sessions seemed to be running smoothly and the therapist did not feel she needed to present this client in clinical supervision.

Towards the end of the sixth session, Hannah said to the therapist, "I love you. You are so kind, just like my grandma". The therapist had unconsciously slipped into the position of benign caregiver. Hannah's transference in that moment was that the therapist was put into the position of the caring, loving, interested Grandma. The therapist's countertransference was that she felt loved. A need that was unmet in her own childhood.

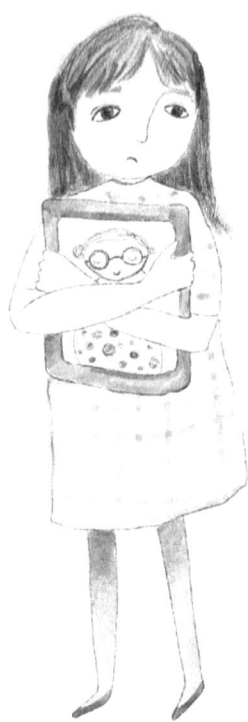

Figure 5.1 Hannah.

Here we have a clear example of positive countertransference. Hannah saw the therapist as caring, wise, and empathetic, all beneficial for the therapeutic process. Had this (counter)transference been missed, a reexperiencing of profound loss would have inevitably happened. Through clinical supervision, the therapist was able to utilise her own countertransference to support Hannah through her journey of grief. Most importantly, Hannah was able to experience a symbolic repair© through a positive ending.

Please Leave Your Nervous System at the Door!

Let's think about the following scenarios that you may have experienced of in therapy sessions:

- suddenly overwhelmed with tiredness, eyelids heavy. Resisting the urge to curl into a ball and doze off?
- experience an irrepressible desire to shout out for your client to stop playing/ talking/moving. Feeling like it is too much and wishing the clock would move faster so you could leave the session?

- become filled with guilt at the realisation that you have been making a mental shopping list rather than focusing on what your client has been doing?
- writing up your notes and realising you remember very little from the session?

You are not alone. These scenarios happen to us all! Regardless of clinical experience, this may occur with even the most dynamic of clients, causing us to feel deep shame and thoughts of how we are failing them. We may dedicate anxious hours employing our scrambled brains to try and work out what happened and what we should do next. Often, we seek new approaches or strategies in response to imposter syndrome, the bully raising its head. Reverting to well-thumbed textbooks we may try and understand why repeated reactions with the same clients occur. Dreading our next session and worrying that we will be unable to perform as a "proper" therapist should.

These experiences are all examples of somatic countertransference. Also referred to as embodied countertransference or body-centred countertransference. This process involves the therapist experiencing the physical state of the client during the session. Let's think about the scenarios through the ANS 'A' States:

- In the session where your body wanted to sleep, were you moving towards a Dorsal State, your nervous system working to AVOID the signals being communicated? How does this physical response link to your client's experience and what they are working through?
- Is it possible that during your clock watching session when you wanted to shout "Stop! Enough!" your system was feeling ALARM and becoming mobilised? Was your client moving into an activated position?
- Which brain regions were available to you during the session you have no notes for? Might your system have moved into AVOID protecting you from becoming energetically enmeshed with your client's perceived threat signals?

Typically, therapists have a good enough understanding of transference and countertransference but may be less familiar with the somatic elements to these processes. Somatic countertransference is positioned as embodied, physical manifestations in the therapist's body. The therapist FEELS what the client feels. We know that children operate from a sensorimotor, bottom-up developmental position. Any experience of early trauma or stressful events that have not been integrated will be expressed and experienced through the body rather than through cognitive understanding or language. Somatic countertransference is the most effective way for our clients to share with us how they experience the world through their body. Indeed, Stone in his 2006 study "The analyst's body as tuning fork", identified that when working with a client who has experienced childhood trauma it is likely somatic reactions in a therapist will occur.

Of course, this intersubjective process does not limit itself to the therapy room. Humans are hardwired to experience the pleasure, pain, distress, and excitement of others. We implicitly understand the 'sameness' of another human because we literally embody their actions, feelings, emotions and sensations. The discovery of the Mirror Neuron System (MNS) in the late 1980's by a team of neuroscientists from the University of Parma provided an additional neurobiological dimension to our understanding of empathy, social identification, and attunement. Investigations showed mirror neurons present in the ventral premotor cortex in macaque monkeys. Results demonstrated that "they fire not only when a monkey is performing an action .... but also, when the monkey passively observes a similar action performed by another" (Cook *et al.*, 2014). In other words, the MNS involves neurons that fire in the brain both when a person performs an action and when they observe the same action performed by someone else.

Further research by Neuroscientist V.S. Ramachandran in the 1990's, showed the connection between phantom limb pain and mirror neurons. Vittorio Gallese, one of the scientists who discovered MNS explains how a common underlying functional mechanism of the MNS is *embodied simulation*, which "mediates our capacity to share the meaning of actions, intentions, feelings, and emotions" (2009).

Having an awareness of the process of somatic countertransference helps us move away from judgemental and unhelpful thinking such as "what am I doing wrong?" or "what is going on with me?" and gives us a whole new perspective, "wow I have an understanding of what my client is feeling!" Sometimes this realisation comes to us in the moment. By taking time to reorganise our internal states and step back into a vagally mediated position, we can consider whether our sensations are shared experiences. Other times, it is less clear.

Let's remind ourselves of Tom's history. From conception, Tom was exposed to toxic stress. At birth, he was placed in the special care baby unit for 6 days. Sally was unable to offer him the necessary buffering needed to counter the stress experienced. For his first 5 months of life with Sally, he received inconsistent care, neglect and was left alone during the frequent, terrifying visits his father made to their home. Tom did not experience a soothed ANS due to a lack of co-regulation from Sally.

In Tom's early sessions, the therapist would find themselves dysregulated, working hard to anchor within the action and activation. Tom would always leap into role play from the moment he entered the playroom, inviting the therapist to battle with his chosen puppet, taking on the challenge of good vs evil. No matter how well prepared the therapist felt, within 5 minutes they would feel exhausted, completely overwhelmed and wanting the play to stop. It felt as if they were being forced back into a trauma loop of action against their will.

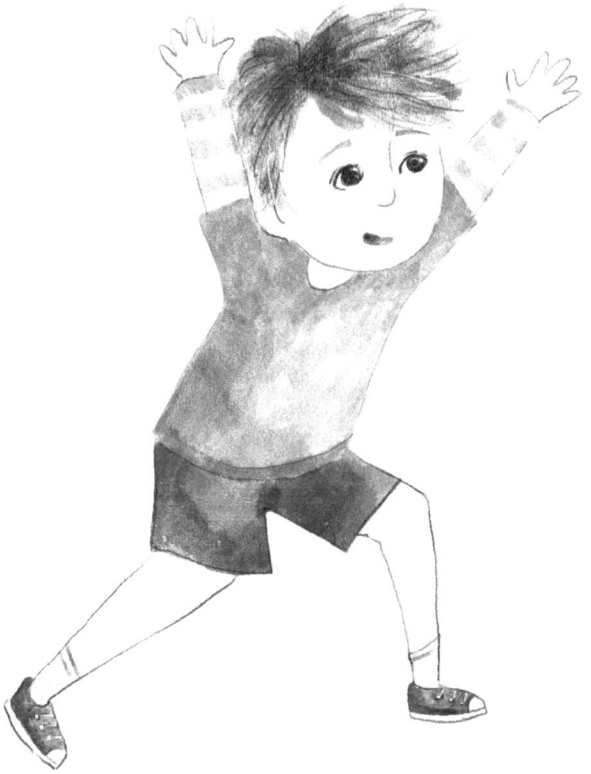

Figure 5.2 Tom.

As a baby it is likely Tom was in an ALARM State: hypervigilant, hyper-aroused, overwhelmed. Aged 7 years, Tom was showing the therapist that he was stuck in an involuntary physiological trauma loop, active, electric, ready to fight. The therapist's somatic countertransference informed them that the activated play was static and post-traumatic. In the here and now, the therapist experienced Tom's body as tired and overwhelmed by his unconscious drive that mobilization equals survival. Superficially, Tom needed to be active. Through the process of somatic countertransference, the therapist understood that Tom needed titrated support to move through The Needs Paradox® and experience social engagement as safe.

As therapists, we expect and are ready to hold dysregulation in others. Many of the children we work with will present with protective, activated nervous systems. In response, much of the time, we will remain regulated, utilising our social engagement system to offer connection, empathy, and communication as a protective response to their dysregulation. Sometimes, just as our clients will have an involuntary response to perceptions of threat so will we. There will inevitably be moments where we are pushed outside of our window of tolerance and our ability to connect will be disrupted.

Coined by Daniel Siegel in 1999, the concept of 'Window of Tolerance' is widely used to consider the range of intensities of emotion that a person can comfortably experience, process, and integrate. Siegel considers that we all have a unique zone of optimal arousal, within which we have full cognitive function and, can think and interact in a way that will allow us to cope with stressors and triggers. If we are outside our Window of Tolerance, we either move into the upper boundary zone of 'hyper-arousal' or below the lower boundary zone of 'hypo-arousal'. Linking this concept to the Polyvagal Theory, we can understand that the optimal arousal zone correlates with the Social Engagement System (AWAKE State); hyper-arousal with the Sympathetic System (ALARM State) and hypo-arousal with the Dorsal Vagal System (AVOID State). Figure 5.3 illustrates this.

It is important to remember that our Window of Tolerance is not set in stone. It can change from moment to moment and will be heavily influenced by physiology (feeling tired, hungry, or unwell) and stress levels. These fluctuations will either extend or diminish our Window of Tolerance, which in turn will impact on how well we are able to tolerate others' dysregulation.

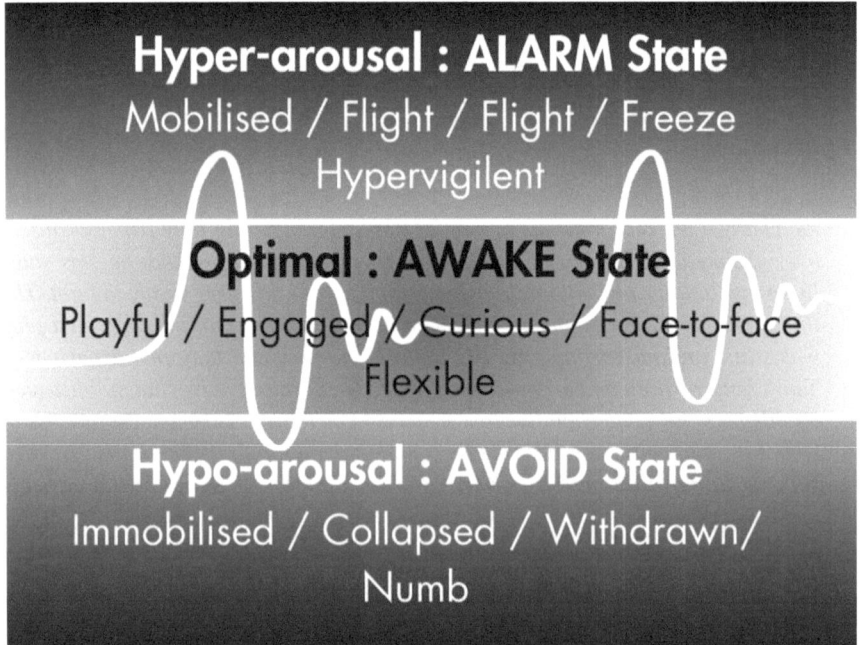

Figure 5.3 ANS 'A' States and arousal.

Creative Activities: Introduction to Your ANS

Activity: Where Have I Journeyed Today?

This activity will give you a moment to reflect on your ANS's journey, before commencing clinical work. Therapists don't simply 'appear' in their clinical space. We journey to get to work and have interactions with people along the way, manage households, look after others, and join the humdrum of humanity. Even working virtually, events and moments will have happened causing fluctuations, expanding, or contracting your Window of Tolerance, and moving you into different autonomic states.

Instructions

Recall nine interactions and events which have taken place from waking until the point you arrive in your therapy space (face-to-face or online). Write these in the boxes along the horizontal axis 'Interactions and Events'. Put a corresponding cross on the vertical axis 'ANS 'A' States' to indicate which State you journeyed to and your level of activation (Figure 5.4).

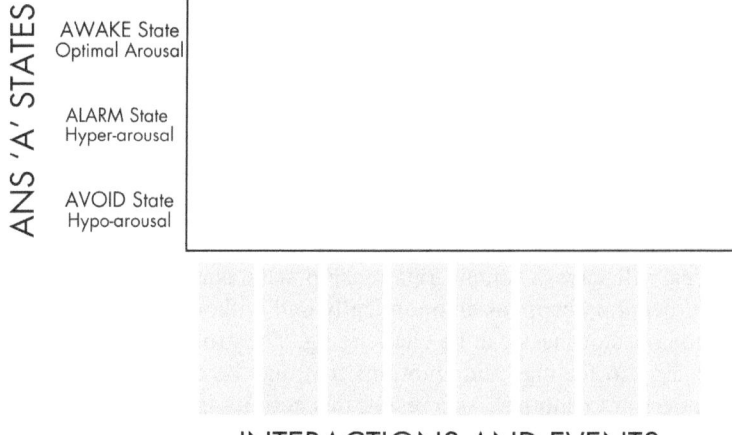

INTERACTIONS AND EVENTS

Figure 5.4 Blank map your day.

In Figure 5.5, we have given you an example of a therapist's morning before getting to work:

Using this simple activity, we can already start to get a picture of how moment to moment interactions can influence our ANS States. Before the therapist came to work, their nervous system had already been moving up and down on the vertical axis through the autonomic states. Their physiology responding to the environment by bringing energy, reducing energy, preparing itself to take on perceived threat. On arrival to work, their system was in hyper-arousal ALARM State.

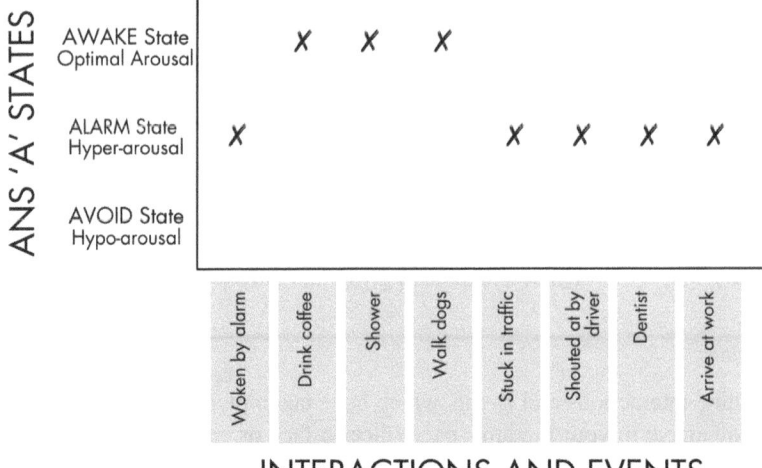

Figure 5.5 Example map your day.

Their heartrate and body temperature increased. Neurologically higher perceptions and thoughts would be inhibited, with the brain favouring more basic somatic and sensory input. It is likely that without grounding, the therapist would not be present in the 'here and now' with regulatory capacity compromised, influencing their ability to offer co-regulation to their first client.

Activity: Becoming Familiar with Your ANS 'A' States

Each of us will have a unique relationship with our own autonomic states. Since neuroception happens autonomically and without our awareness, bringing this to consciousness can be challenging. The process is visceral and sensorial, leading to feelings and emotions that may be uncomfortable, differing from one person to another. As a result, this activity invites you to bring these states to awareness using metaphor. This will grant easier access to the unconscious processes.

Instructions

Please have three pieces of paper and some coloured pens or pencils available. As we take you through the tasks, notice if it is easier or harder for you to access a particular State. Have a curiosity about how familiar this position is to you. Whether or not you have the experience of strongly resisting movement into a protective state. This activity is designed to be offered in the order given to ensure that we leave you in the AWAKE State of 'okayness'. If you choose to use these exercises with clients, please ensure you do the same.

ALARM State

We are going to start by exploring the ALARM State. Bring to mind a character from a film or TV show that is in sympathetic activation. This character will have a body filled with too much energy, prepared for action, ready to protect itself. What do you notice about the character's behaviour?

In *Column 1*, write down the character's traits. Next, choose a colour to represent these traits and behaviours. Represent this in *Column 2* through line and shape. As you sit with this image, have curiosity about moments when you have felt this image seep into your body. What does your body *feel* like to be in this State? Do you notice any *sensations* in your body? Where do you notice these *sensations* in your body? How do your muscles feel? What do you notice about your *breathing*? Make a note of these sensations in *Column 3*.

Create an image to represent how your internal State feels. Give it a name. Now, let us consider what may have set a sympathetic flow of energy in motion. Be curious about what brought this energy to your body. Did something happen to you? Did something happen within the environment? Did you hear, see, touch, smell, taste something? Did you have a thought? Mark these down in *Column 4* through words or images. Now, listen to your body as it tells you what it needs you to do to move back to the AWAKE State. Do you need to stretch, move, breathe deeply, close your eyes, move your face, or smile? Do you need to get a drink? Do you need to move to a different space? Pay attention and respond to these needs, taking as much time as is necessary. Write down in *Column 5* what was needed from yourself, the environment, and another to return to a position of 'okayness' (Figure 5.6).

1.Character Traits	2. Colour, Line, Shape	3.Bodily Sensations	4. What has brought you here?	5. What do you need to do?
• jumpy • tearful • shouts • shaking • anxious • suspicious • frightened	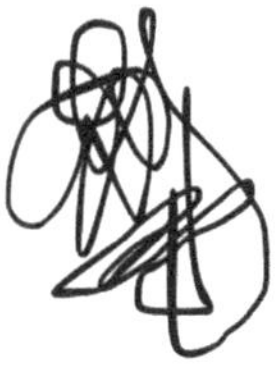 Squibble	• short breath • cold • heart racing • tight chest • can't hear anything • electricity in stomach 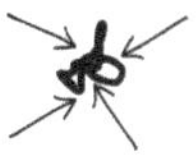	• unsmiling faces • being ignored • loud sudden noises • fear of failure	• walk outside • receive a smile • breathe • pull shoulders back • move head and neck

Figure 5.6 Explorations of ALARM State.

AVOID State

We invite you to explore the Dorsal Vagal: AVOID State. When you are ready, close your eyes for a moment. Focus on your heart rate. Consider whether you need to slow your breathing and move into more meditative quieter state. When you feel that your body has slowed down, gently open your eyes. Now, we would like you to remember the last time you gave yourself permission to take a 'Duvet Day'. Looking back to this moment, what did your body want to do? Did you need to lie down and listen to music or binge on a box set? Did you go to bed and withdraw? Did you turn off your phone, cancel an appointment, or shut yourself in?

Take a piece of paper and the pens/pencils. Represent this experience in the middle of the page through colour, line, or shape. It might be abstract, or you might create a character. There is no right or wrong as to how you represent your image.

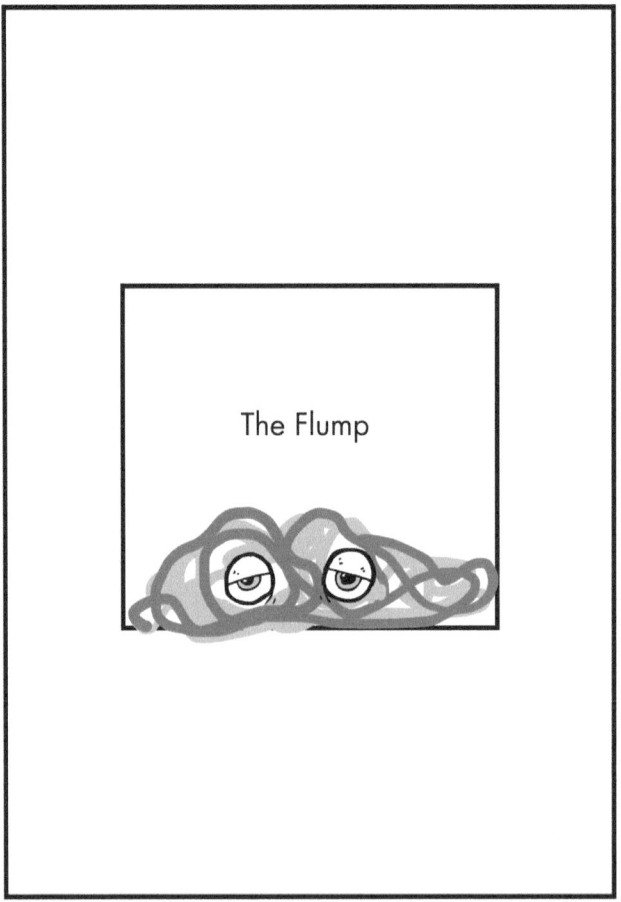

Figure 5.7 Part 1. AVOID State.

Does your image have a name? If so, write it down. We would like you to consider what brought you to the AVOID State. Write down all the different things at the top of the page.

Stepping into the AVOID State may have changed your energy which will be circulating in your system. Take a moment to notice what you need to move gently to sympathetic and mobilisation. Focusing on the here and now, notice what your body needs to re-energise your ANS. When you are ready, move your body in whichever way it needs; you choose. Once you have noticed a state shift change, return to a comfortable space, and check in with yourself. When you are ready, on the same piece of paper, write down the different ways that supported you to connect back to self.

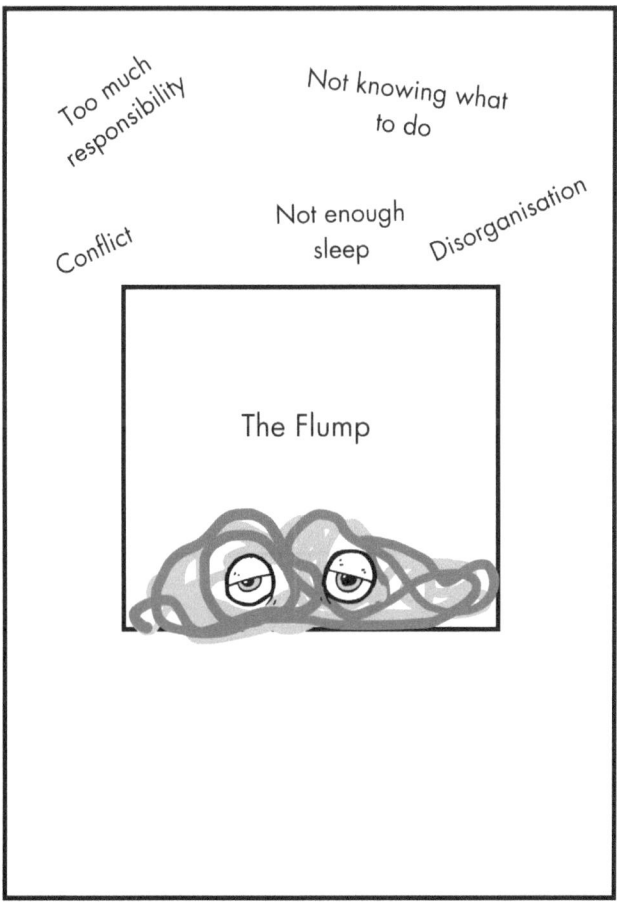

Figure 5.8 Part 2. AVOID State.

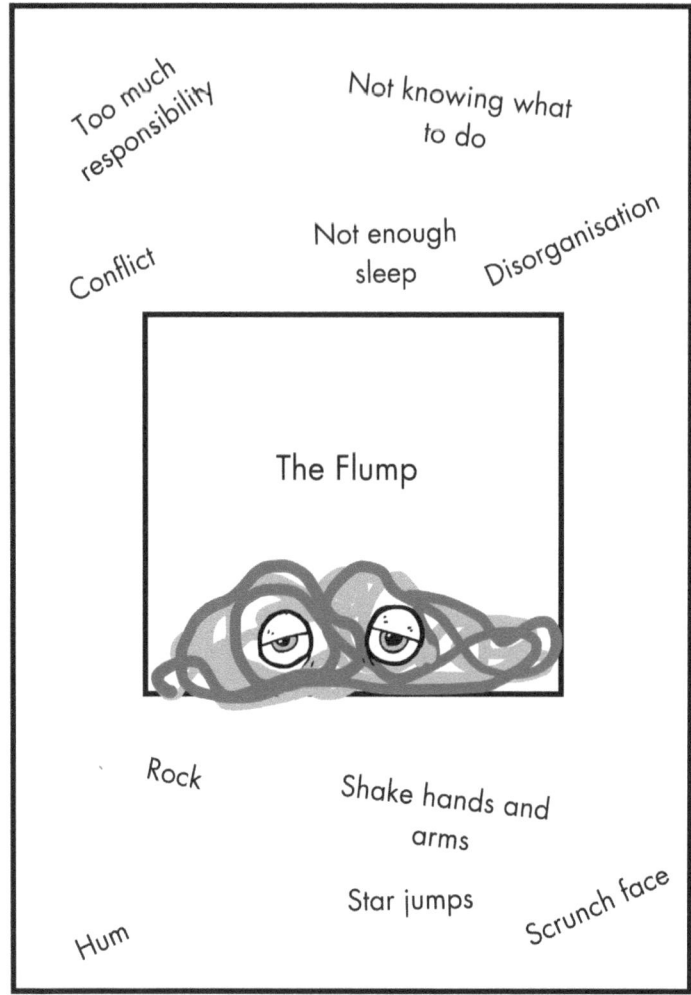

Too much responsibility

Not knowing what to do

Conflict

Not enough sleep

Disorganisation

The Flump

Rock

Shake hands and arms

Star jumps

Scrunch face

Hum

Figure 5.9 Part 3. AVOID State.

AWAKE State

This is your final destination, your AWAKE State. When you are in this position, you are in a vagally mediated State, you are 'home'. In the AWAKE State, you have an easy connection with people. You can laugh, think, write reports, respond to difficulties, and have a generalised sense that the world is okay.

When you are ready, bring to mind an animal that represents the AWAKE State. What is the animal doing? What do you think the animal's attitude to the world is? How does this animal respond to others?

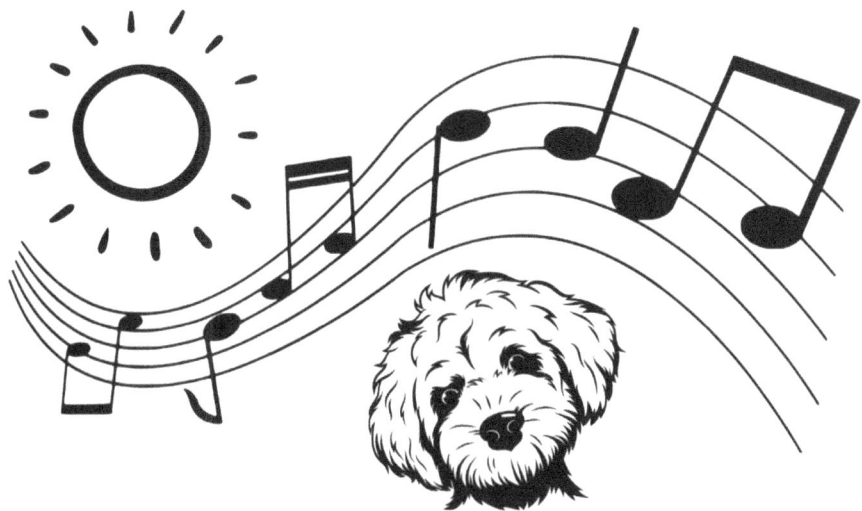

Figure 5.10 Exploration of AWAKE State.

Connecting symbolically to the animal, we encourage you to be the animal for a few minutes and be curious about the experience. When do you feel like this animal? As the animal, where are you right now? Are you alone or with others? What are you doing? What conditions does the animal need from itself, the environment and others to feel comfortable and safe? On your final piece of paper, create an image which illustrates all that you need to feel ok.

Next, place all three pictures in front of you and consider the following questions:

1   Which ANS State was the easiest for your body to move into?
2   How much did you embody this State?
3   As you immersed yourself in this State, was it a familiar experience?
4   Look at the images in front of you and focus on the ALARM State and the AVOID State. Consider what you wrote for both these States and the energy that brought you to them. Does anything in these images relate to any moments in your therapy room in relation to a client and you? Have any of the experiences within these two images happened to you in the therapy room?
5   Consider what you needed to do when in these States to move towards a generalised sense of connection and safety. Are there elements that you can utilise to support your AWAKE State either before, during or after therapy sessions? Do you need to take time to integrate more connected energy into your day?

The purpose of this activity was to help you to begin to think about your nervous system through the lens of hierarchy and ANS 'A' States. As a therapist, this activity can assist you to formulate an understanding of why you might move into a position of ALARM or AVOID with your clients. Having a recognition of our generalised triggers is hugely important and with intentionality can support the ability to predict and prepare for moments that may present with particular clients or referral needs. This expansion of self-awareness supports higher vagal tone development which in in turn leads to greater moment to moment regulatory capacity.

Emotional Regulator

Working with children invites non-verbal, bidirectional communication of the mind and body. Through their body, clients unconsciously transmit to us their true feeling States, relational expectations, and perceptions of adults. To act as the emotional regulator for our clients we need to have full access to our social engagement system. When this is available, we can see the bigger picture. We are more curious and flexible having connection to our own experiences. In addition, we have empathy for ourselves and our clients whilst experiencing and processing our thoughts and emotions simultaneously. As a socially engaged therapist we are aware of the present moment, anchored in the here and now, reacting in ways that make sense for the situation that we are in. When we are able to move through the different ANS 'A' States bringing matched energy and action when needed, we can tolerate our client's feelings as they move through The Needs Paradox®.

Chapter 6

Perceptions of Play and Metaphor

Children of all ages express their realities through play and metaphors. This form of communication is a vehicle that is more familiar and comfortable as "play allows children to put into words, the words of play" (Barnes, 2013).

In this chapter we explore the realms of play and metaphor which are intricate facets and shape our understanding of ourselves and the universe in which we live. Play is crucial in childhood development, serving as a means through which children explore the world around them and learn about social relationships. Similarly, metaphor plays a crucial role in shaping our perspectives and understanding of the world. In essence, both offer unique insights into the complexities of human experience through processes of creativity imagination, and meaning-making.

Play

It is difficult to find a concise, clear, and agreed definition of play. Else (2009) suggests that "play is the way humans develop efficient brains" and that it benefits the development of bodies, relationships, and minds.

Stevens (2014) asserts that "there are clearly defined functions for play in evolution and neurobiological development, which range from practicing survival skills to developing higher-order thinking, such as imagination, pattern recognition, metacognition, empathy, and creative thinking". Moreover, play creates opportunities to develop social skills, self-regulation, and a responsive nervous system to life (Wheeler & Dillman Taylor, 2016).

Kestly (2014) explains that play accepts the child's memories and experiences without judgement, and in the process of play new synapses are created as new energy and information can fundamentally rewrite them, resulting in behaviour change or different coping mechanisms.

Metaphor

The use of metaphor is supported by Sunderland (2000) who states that stories and metaphors are "more respectful and far less invasive" as they speak to the child at a deeper and more meaningful level, helping them to process and understand their situation at a safe and contained distance from reality.

DOI: 10.4324/9781003412571-7

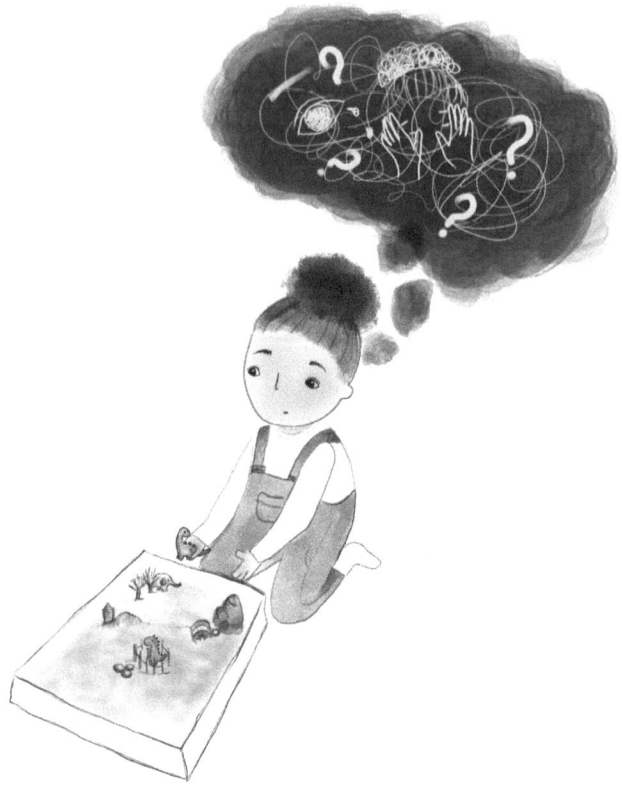

Figure 6.1 Play and metaphor.

Gardner and Harper (1997) explain that the metaphors and images that are present in children's play help the child to distinguish their imagination and inner conflicts from their outer reality. Reminding us that this is why the use of metaphor and narrative is so powerful for change and healing.

Working with metaphors and symbols in play therapy are milestones of Jungian approach. Children use metaphors and symbols in their drawing, sand play and so on, to connect with their unconscious. Therapists who apply the Jungian approach, trust that the process of the unconscious makes meaning of metaphors for the child.

Child Development

Several child development theories emphasise the significance of play in children's growth, learning, and socialisation. Multifaceted, play is important in cognitive, social, emotional, and cultural aspects of child development. Many highlight the importance of play including the following:

Theorist	Concept	Summary of contribution to child development
John Bowlby	Attachment Theory	Focuses on the importance of early relationships in shaping children's socioemotional development
Jean Piaget	Theory of Cognitive Development	Describes how children construct their understanding of the world through interaction with their environment. Identified play as a primary mechanism through which children explore and make sense of their surroundings.
Lev Vygotsky	Sociocultural Theory	Emphasised the social and cultural context of learning and development. Suggests that children's cognitive development is influenced by social interactions and social tools.
Eric Erikson	Psychosocial Theory	Proposed that individuals go through a series of states each characterised by specific developmental tasks and conflicts.

Neurobiological Perspective of Play and Metaphor

From a neurobiological perspective, play and metaphor allow the child to revisit implicit memories which impact on a sense of self and interactions in the present with "a unique role in accessing and remapping lower brain regions" (Goodyear-Brown, 2019). The use of non-verbal mediums in therapy is supported by evidence in the field of neuroscience, as is the notion that it is possible that "a corrective emotional experience in which old patterns of relating can be replaced with new more healthy patterns" (Cadogan, 2016). For this reason, Landreth (2002) suggests that "play is the symbolic language of self-expression, a way of working out balance and control in their lives", with Barnes (2013) describing metaphor as symbols which "have a greater meaning than their outward image".

During early child development, nerve cells in the brain undergo synaptogenesis. This process is characterised by rapid growth and extensive branching of dendrites with the formation of connections between neurons. Play is essential in these processes as it has a significant role in shaping the brain's architecture. Professor Huberman: Neuroscientist and Ophthalmologist (2022), suggests that play engages the process of neural connections in the brain and that emotions create neural pathways through behaviour. If pathways are not taken, they disappear, however, play will continue to strengthen the remaining connections. Seemingly, at around the age of 25 years, approximately 40% of brain neurons will disappear through a biological process of pruning whilst connections that remain are strengthened by becoming thicker and robust as "cells that fire together, wire together" (Shatz, 1992).

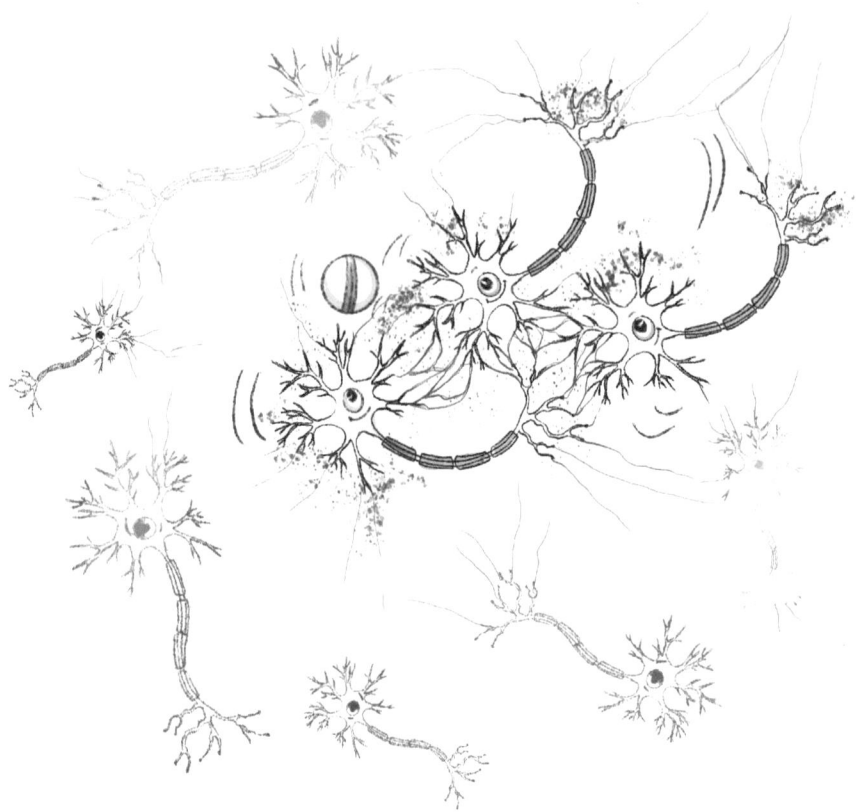

Figure 6.2 Play and the brain.

At a basic level it is often thought the right hemisphere of the brain is "connected to emotions" (Ammann, 1991). We have also come to understand that the right hemisphere is involved in processing emotions and regulating emotional responses. However, it is now acknowledged that both the left and right hemispheres are differentially involved in processing emotions. Research suggests that play is embedded deep in the circuitry of the brain and is key to neuroplasticity, influencing various neural pathways and networks associated with learning, emotional regulation, social interaction, and sensorimotor integration.

We know that play activates the brain's reward pathways including the release of neurotransmitters such as dopamine, serotonin, and endorphins. According to Professor Andrew Huberman (2022) play stimulates the brain stem to release endogenous opioids which are self-made biological opioids that support body relaxation including posture, soft eyes, and head tilts. Opioids alongside the mode of play provide opportunities for the pre-frontal cortex to notice, explore, and expand our capacity to interact in the space within and between. This opens new ways of being in different contexts. These processes are crucial for the child to develop executive functioning; anticipation, regulating emotions, planning, decision making, whole brain integration. Additionally, play lowers cortisol, increasing dopamine, oxytocin and gamma-aminobutyric acid (GABA) which support brain neuroplasticity. It is worth noting that the body and brain can only engage in play when there are low amounts of adrenaline (epinephrine) as too much will inhibit play.

Neurotransmitter	Role
Gamma-aminobutyric acid (GABA)	Primary inhibitory neurotransmitter in the central nervous system. Reduces neuronal excitability throughout the nervous system.
Dopamine	Associated with pleasure, reward, motivation.
Endorphins	Act as natural painkillers and mood enhancers. Released in response to stress and pain, as-well as during activities including exercise and pain.

In the context of psychology and neuroscience, the study of emotions is wide ranging with no one concept being agreed upon. Jaak Panksepp, Neuroscientist and Psychobiologist, spent much of his career researching and understanding mammalian emotions from primal operating systems embedded in neural circuitry. Panksepp coined the term 'affective neuroscience' mapping seven biological primary emotions across the mammalian brain (1998). He provided data to show the existence of seven instinctive emotional-motivational systems in the midbrain of mammals and humans (Panksepp, 2003, 2007) which are genetically inherited and independent of experience or cognitions as follows:

Emotional system	Behaviour
Seeking	Core emotional-motivational circuit which is the foundation of all emotional processes. Motivates exploration, curiosity, and search for resources. Associated with feelings of anticipation and excitement. Crucial in learning.
Rage/Anger	Involved in responses to frustration, threat, or challenge. Can manifest as aggressive or defensive behaviours. Is crucial for self-preservation.
Fear	Responsible for detection and response to potential threats in the environment. Triggers the fight or flight response to avoid danger.
Lust	Associated with reproductive behaviours and the pursuit of sexual gratification. Drives mating behaviours and facilitates the continuation of the species.
Care/Bonding	Relates to nurturing and caregiving behaviours, particularly in parental care. Promotes attachment, bonding, and social connection.

Emotional system	Behaviour
Panic/Grief	Activated in response to separation from attachment figures or the loss of social bonds. Produces distress and motivates efforts to restore social connections.
Play/Social	Involved in social play behaviours and interactions that promote bonding and social cohesion. Facilitates learning, socialisation, and the development of social skills.

Psychiatrist and Neuroscientist, Dr. Bruce Perry has extensively studied the impact of early experiences, including play on brain development and mental health. He developed the Neurosequential Model of Therapeutics (NMT, 2006) emphasising the critical role of relational interactions and supportive environments in shaping children's neural circuitry and overall well-being. An integrated approach to sequencing neurodevelopment, it considers how the brain develops in response to experiences, especially traumatic ones, thus interventions can be tailored and titrated accordingly. The essence of NMT lies in its in understanding of the interconnectedness between brain development, relational experiences, and the impact of trauma. The approach recognises that the brain develops in a sequential manner, with different areas and systems maturing at different rates. This sequential development influences how individuals respond to their environment, process information, and regulate emotions.

Understanding that play is a natural and spontaneous behaviour, Perry (2006) suggests that it is a fundamental mechanism through which children learn about themselves and the world, developing social skills and resilience. NMT recognises the therapeutic value of play and creative expression in promoting neural integration, emotional regulation, and healing. The approach encourages the incorporation of playful and creative interventions to help children regain regulation through somatosensory activities from which safety emerges (Gaskill & Perry, 2014). Activities could include, drawing, music, dance and movement, breathing, relaxation, walking. Once regulation and safety are achieved children can connect to relational aspects of child therapy.

Polyvagal Theory and Play

The Polyvagal Theory suggests that social play allows the blending of the parasympathetic and the sympathetic nervous systems without triggering protective responses. Blending the AWAKE State with the ALARM State, or the AWAKE State and the AVOID State during play requires the child to detect a neuroception of safety, which communicates that they are 'just' playing.

Children's autonomic nervous systems undergo significant development and maturation from infancy. Their bodies and the autonomic nervous system are intricately connected, each having vital roles in regulating in various bodily functions and responses. Gradually, as children grow and develop, the regulatory mechanism of the ANS becomes more refined.

A lot of children that we work with have not had cues of safety. Instead, they will have experienced repeated cues of danger, impacting their behaviour which may indicate that they are experiencing stress, fear, and anxiety. Manifesting in various ways, behaviours may include:

- Aggression or acting out
- Withdrawal or isolation
- Hyperactivity or Impulsivity
- Avoidance
- Regression
- Hypervigilance
- Emotional outbursts
- Difficulty with transitions

Feelings can be overwhelming with an autonomic response of mobilisation or immobilisation. Although Porges' work on the ANS and Social Engagement System does not focus primarily on play and play behaviour, it offers a valuable framework for understanding the physiological mechanisms underlying social behaviour, emotion regulation, and interpersonal interactions. Recognising that these are all closely linked to principles of the Polyvagal Theory, play can promote the activation of the Ventral Vagal Complex associated with states of calm, social engagement, and connection.

Play can only occur when the child perceives that they are safe. In the context of play and the Polyvagal Theory, it can be applied to understand how play experiences influence the nervous system and social engagement. With emphasis on safety, social engagement, co-regulation and emotional regulation, the therapeutic nature of play can create an understanding of brain-body connection. In addition, play enables the child to experience increased levels of excitement or tension without triggering the body's stress response mechanism.

The body serves as a vehicle for emotional expression during play. Children may use their body language, facial expressions, and vocalisations to convey their emotions while engaging in pretend play or interactive games. This embodiment of emotions enriches the play experience helping them to understand and regulate their feelings. Erik Erikson observed that "to play out is the most natural self-healing measure childhood affords" (1963).

When applying the framework of the Polyvagal Theory to the intersection of play we can consider the three organising principles, neuroception, hierarchy, and co-regulation to inform our work.

Neuroception

Neuroception is crucial in determining whether an environment is perceived as safe for play. When the autonomic nervous system detects cues of safety and trust, children are more likely to engage in social play, such as co-operative games or imaginative play. These conditions influence the autonomic nervous system's response to playful stimuli, helping to regulate arousal levels during play. If the child perceives the environment as safe and enjoyable, neuroception promotes parasympathetic activation, leading to a state of relaxation and receptivity to playful experiences.

Conversely, if the environment is perceived as threatening or unpredictable, neuroception may trigger defensive responses, inhibiting playful behaviour. This will promote mobilisation: Fight or flight or immobilisation: collapse.

Through neuroception, the body responds with either 'matched' or 'mismatched' energy (Dana, 2018). Matched neuroception reflects an appropriate response and energy to effectively manage the situation. Once the feeling of danger is over, there is a return to homeostasis. Mismatched neuroception reflects inadequate energy to respond to the situation. This can result in too much energy, the ALARM State or too little energy, the AVOID State. As the child plays or uses metaphor, the hope is that there is matched energy and that they can return to homeostasis.

Teddy lived with his mum, Jemma until he was aged 18 months. There was lack of opportunity to play with his mum and there were very few toys. When Teddy arrives for his play therapy sessions, he runs into the room and is chaotic, throwing toys and shouting at the therapist. Boundaries are put in place by the therapist and Teddy flops and curls into a ball. Here we see Teddy has moved from an ALARM State where there is too much energy into the AVOID State where there is too little energy. Despite the therapist providing the core conditions and responsive attunement, Teddy's felt sense of safety is compromised with perceived threat leading to mismatched neuroception within the context of therapy.

Hierarchy

Play interacts with the autonomic nervous system's hierarchical responses in several ways. According to Kestly (2014) the Polyvagal Theory provides a lens from which play can be seen through the ANS. Stephen Porges suggests that play is a 'neural exercise' which is crucial in shaping experiences and behaviour enhancing the co-regulation of physiological states. In the process of play there is a moving back and forth between autonomic states. In essence, the window of tolerance expands, moving the child from a state of fear into social engagement.

Social play affords the blending of the parasympathetic and sympathetic nervous systems which creates opportunities for states of heightened arousal without triggering a defensive (mobilised) response (Porges, 2011). However, we must remember that parasympathetic, sympathetic, and dorsal vagal are pathways in service of survival. Responses to a neuroception of threat work in a specified order and can only be moved through in sequence. The child may move between all three pathways many times over the course of a therapy session. Porges (2011) suggests that "the difference between the fight/flight and play is that while mobilizing, we're making eye contact and engaging each other". As therapists, we diffuse the cues of threat with social cues utilising the sympathetic nervous system to support movement without moving into defensive fight/flight behaviours.

The Social Engagement System is mediated by the myelinated vagus nerve and operates optimally in states of safety and perceived social connection. Physiologically, play occurs when the Ventral Vagal System is activated, and the sympathetic system is mobilised to create a state that supports mobilised play without fear (Porges, 2011). This allows the child to engage in adventurous, active, and imaginative play whilst feeling safe and connected. On the other hand, play can also be experienced as immobilisation without fear when the dorsal vagal system is activated in the presence of safety. This allows the child to experience and manage low states of arousal whilst continuing to play without fear of harm.

Co-regulation

Co-regulation is a biological imperative of reciprocal regulation of our autonomic states. Play and co-regulation are interconnected. Through play, the child can engage in co-regulatory behaviours, mirroring, attunement, and empathy which support the activation of the AWAKE State which promotes feelings of safety and connection. In the experience of co-regulation, the therapist's nervous system will influence the child's nervous system to foster feelings of connection, safety, and trust. As an interactive process, there will be a reciprocal sending and receiving of signals of safety with each regulating the other in the process.

Hannah has a secure attachment foundation with her parents. She is struggling to come to terms with her grandmother's death and was often tearful. The therapist has gently fostered a climate of empathy, compassion and understanding to help Hannah process the loss of her grandmother. Hannah has entered her therapy in an AWAKE State. She has engaged within the therapeutic relationship and through co-regulation, has used metaphor and play to express and process some of her thoughts and feelings. Her parents report that she is less tearful and that most nights she is going to sleep without waking. Claire reports that Hannah is not routinely coming into her bed overnight which was one of the goals of therapy.

To summarise, hierarchy determines that if the ANS experiences the environment as safe and supportive, the body will activate the AWAKE State mediated by the ventral vagal complex. With feelings of safety, connection, and trust, the child will use their facial expressions, voice prosody, eye contact, and body to engage in play and playful activities.

If the child senses cues of danger, there is often an intense reaction in their bodies moving them into a sympathetic ALARM State with the possible risk of moving into dorsal vagal, the AVOID State.

Vagal Brake

As discussed in Chapter 3 the vagal brake is essential in maintaining physiological homeostasis by modulating the heart rate. It is also involved in regulating emotional responses by increasing vagal tone.

Play and the vagal brake are interconnected. Through the neural exercise of play, the vagal brake can be 'fine-tuned' which supports the co-regulation of physiological states (Porges, 2017). As we consider the ANS 'A' states, we see that the AWAKE State engages the vagal brake and social engagement behaviours. Play can be characterised by either high or low states of arousal because of the blending of the parasympathetic and sympathetic nervous systems. Whether the child's play is active or calm we see that there is high social engagement from the child with the therapist.

When there is the removal of the vagal brake, there is an increase in sympathetic arousal and a move towards the ALARM State or AVOID State. When the child is in the ALARM State, defensive play behaviours of fight, and flight are mobilised. When the child is in the AVOID State, the defensive play of immobilisation is activated with a collapse response. In either of these states, the play is stuck or stagnant characterised by an inactive social engagement system. Usually, the child plays compulsively, and they are not aware of the therapist's presence. Indeed, what we find is that there is a lack of imagination, joy, spontaneity, and variety, and that play fails to bring relief (Gil, 2006; Levine & Kline, 2006). From the perspective of the therapist, there is strong countertransference. It seems that the child is re-enacting rather than 'playing', leaving the therapist with a sense of overwhelm.

> *Tom experienced developmental trauma during critical windows of his development. Before accessing therapy, he had not been able to process or integrate his early lived experience. During the initial stages of the therapeutic work, Tom wanted to flight, run out of the room, or hide under the tables. Here we see that Tom was in his ALARM State. His play was defensive and mobilised, likely driven from fear and a neuroception of danger. We can conceptualise that Tom felt threatened or powerless with his defensive play giving him a sense of control. Recently, Tom's play and the way in which he is using metaphors has changed. He is inviting the therapist into his play with lots of collaborative and connected play including metaphorical and imaginative role play, co-operative games and hide and seek. Here we see that Tom is more able to be in his AWAKE State as there is playful and social engagement with the therapist, with the toys and with the environment.*

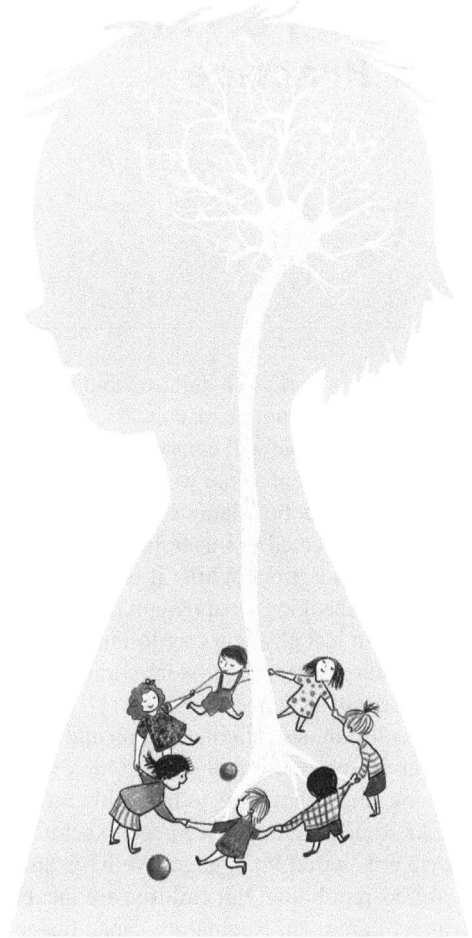

Figure 6.3 Play and regulation.

Child therapy can act as a 'brain sculptor' by releasing chemicals in the brain, creating new neural pathways, and impacting on anatomical structures. Gross (2021) suggests that metaphors are an indirect way of processing, translating the nonliteral into the literal, taking something abstract and invisible, and turning it into something concrete and visible. As therapists, we need to communicate a steady stream of 'play signals' to keep the child within the safety of their autonomic window of tolerance.

Chapter 7

Integrating the Polyvagal Theory into Practice

As child therapists, we come to work with children and young people with all our knowledge and experiences. We are not blank canvasses, and neither are the clients that we work with. In this chapter, we will consider how the foundational concepts of the Polyvagal Theory are pertinent to the work of regulating a child's stress response system through the therapeutic relationship.

In life, staying safe and connected is imperative. From the moment a baby is born, they need safety and connection. Whilst it is possible that certain physical tasks, bathing, dressing, and changing a nappy could be performed by robots, human babies require more than just physical care to thrive. Without another's nervous system, the baby will die. A nervous system without connection to someone else's nervous system is a death sentence.

Throughout human evolution, social connections and co-operation have been essential for survival and reproductive success. Our evolutionary history has shaped our bodies, brains, and behaviours to be highly attuned to social engagement and interaction. As social mammals, we need to acknowledge how our bodies evolved and that we are 'wired' to engage. We have an innate physiological and biological drive for co-regulation, but children are incapable of emotion regulation without a primary caregiver. Regulatory capacities are slowly developed which form brain and nervous system circuitry. Hence, children who have grown up alone, especially those with developmental trauma, often have an inability to inhibit defence responses. This means that the "nervous system is in a continual state of activated mobilization (hyper-aroused) or immobilization (hypo-aroused) survival" (Dana, 2018). Furthermore, the experience of early trauma impacts negatively on the child's view of the world, relationships with others, and their ability to trust.

Although brain scanning (neuroimaging) is in its infancy, some studies have shown that children who have experienced developmental trauma have changes in the structure, volume and shape of the hippocampus, corpus callosum, medial prefrontal cortex. The American Academy of Pediatrics states "the biological response to this toxic stress can be incredibly destructive and last a lifetime" (2014). As a result, a child's 'templates' for managing emotions can be inadequate and their

DOI: 10.4324/9781003412571-8

ways of responding can be ineffective especially in times of crisis and perceived threat. Remembering that we need to honour the body's neurobiology and physiology which always responds in service of survival, we know that "therapy and other healing relationships utilize all levels of connection to alter neural network activation and balance" (Cozolino, 2006). In this landscape of the child who is full of emotional turbulence, the therapist becomes important as a witness and emotional regulator on their journey of physiological homeostasis towards growth, restoration, and healing.

Therapist Self-Awareness

As therapists, an important notion to hold in our mind and in our body is what Polyvagal therapeutic applications might look like for ourselves before we can be more effective in clinical work.

According to Fuchs (2004) "psychotherapy is a unique form of communication among all types of social interactions between two individuals, a client and a therapist". The therapeutic alliance between the therapist and child requires both verbal and non-verbal social interactions. To be an emotional regulator for the client, the therapist needs to have an awareness and understanding of their own felt sense of safety and bi-directional connection from the brain to body to relationally regulate the child's nervous system (Geller & Porges, 2014), a psychobiological core of the therapeutic relationship.

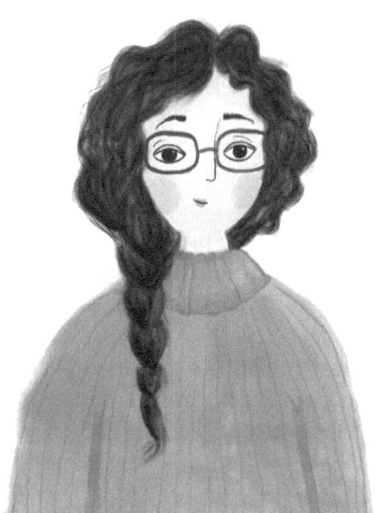

Figure 7.1 Therapist.

Part of this is about identifying one's own limitations regardless of experience. We need to acknowledge our flaws and failures to have a nervous system at ease with playing and creativity, a neural exercise. However, it is mostly about therapist self-awareness which is often supported by the on-going process of personal therapy to gain a depth of understanding of one's own nervous system. According to Jennings (1993) "if we choose to work with damaged children then we must be prepared to acknowledge our own internal damaged child and seek personal therapy for ourselves. If we avoid this, then we are in danger of exploiting the child, of searching for our own resolutions through our work with children".

We also know that therapist self-care is of paramount importance for maintaining wellbeing and preventing burnout. We need to become experts in our own nervous systems which will better equip us to regulate our ANS 'A' States. We often find our window of tolerance challenged by the volume and complexity of our caseloads. We need to give ourselves permission to take our time and say no. Working effectively and ethically requires us to look after ourselves, replenish, and restore. This is true self-care. Additionally, we might engage in daily self-care activities including breath work, yoga, massages, dancing, playing sports, and reading a book. All can reduce heart rate and lower cortisol which may enhance our effectiveness as clinicians. We can then be a healthy playful collaborator by serving as an attuned emotional regulator to the child's nervous system (Schore & Schore, 2008).

Therapist Position

We are guided by different theories and orientations which enrich our work. The Polyvagal Theory emphasises the role of the therapeutic relationship to support regulation of the child's stress response via the vagus nerve. From the perspective of therapists, creative mediums will be part of the 'toolkit' alongside play which as a neural exercise, requires "synchronous and reciprocal behaviours between individuals creating a deepened awareness of each other's social engagement system" (Porges, 2017). Whilst there is a place for cognitive frameworks for working with children and young people, Ryan (2007) suggests that we need to "appreciate the limits of exclusively cognitive approaches for understanding the initiation and regulation of human behaviour".

A therapist 'relationally regulates' a child's nervous system within therapy, which strengthens a child's self-regulation over time (Geller & Porges, 2014). For therapy to be effective the nervous system of a child must detect features of safety in both the therapy environment and the therapist (Porges, 2017).

In respect of clinical work, it is helpful to remember that we are not medical professionals and are interested in how autonomic processes impact emotional and behavioural wellbeing. It is useful to remind ourselves that the vagus nerve travels from the base of the skull all the way through the body, carrying information between the brain and internal organs. A bi-directional nerve when there is homeostasis, the body brain connection is in a healthy state. It is trauma that disconnects the brain from the body as the energy becomes stuck in the nervous system.

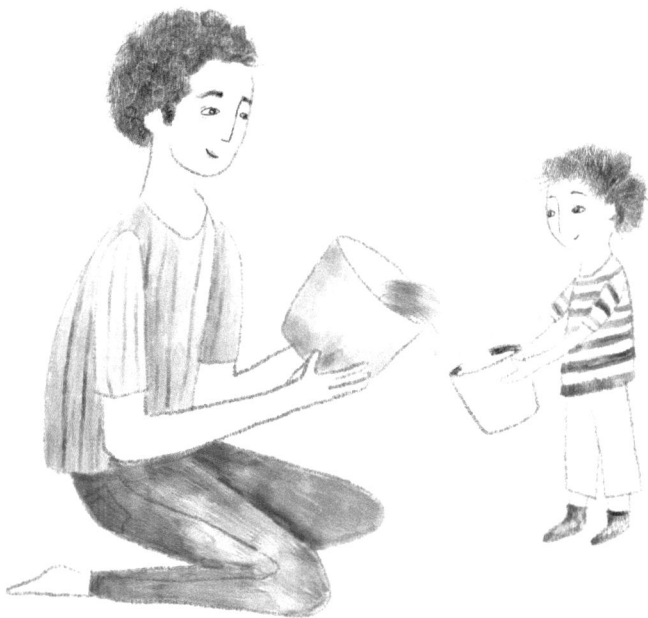

Figure 7.2 Relational regulation.

A Polyvagal Stance (O'Neill & McDonald) and the successful application of theory is not necessarily the capacity to hold all information, rather the ability to sense one's own inner states and those of the client to enhance the therapeutic process. The aim is for the therapist is to have a self-regulatory embodied mind to support the client's aroused states, modifying through the experience of co-regulation for homeostatic functioning. As such, awareness and skill are as important as knowledge and understanding.

The Polyvagal Theory and Physiology of Trauma

Malchiodi (2008) suggests that "in order to help children who have been traumatised, it is first important to have a working knowledge of the physiology of trauma, know how the brain is organised, and understand how the body and mind react to traumatic events". We also see that trauma can impact neuroception leading the child to perceive safety as a threat triggering defensive responses even in non-threatening situations. Therapists understanding of the Polyvagal Theory and conceptualising a neurophysiological map as a way of the child telling their story through their body allows tracking of autonomic states and brain states, tailoring interventions accordingly.

ANS 'A' states		Brain structure	
Dorsal Vagal	Moves us out of connection and co-regulation into immobilisation.	Brainstem	Primitive and oldest part of the brain. Responsible for controlling basic bodily functions, breathing, and heart rate. Instinctively avoids danger.
Sympathetic	Moves us away from connection to protection into mobilisation.	Limbic system	The emotional part of the brain includes the amygdala and hippocampus. Centre of emotions, monitoring, understanding, and building emotional connections whether healthy or unhealthy.
Ventral Vagal	Moves us into connection, co-regulation, and social engagement.	Frontal Lobe/ Prefrontal Cortex	The analytical part of the brain makes sense of feelings, emotions, and situations that occur. Responsible for reflecting on and processing information.

Creating a safe and predictable therapeutic space where we offer embodied responses will encourage the expression of autonomic states. However, a continuum of the approach through a polyvagal lens, regardless of the modality should be based on where the child is at and what they need in the moment and not on how long the session is. This requires therapist flexibility to move between non-directive and directive interventions as they attend to the child's nervous system in any given moment.

Application of the Polyvagal Theory

Children and young people present with behaviours that can often be difficult to make sense of. Based on the innate drive for connection and social engagement, we often see that children's difficulties are because of co-regulation disruptions and that they are struggling with their autonomic states of arousal. Babies and infants are highly attuned to the emotional cues of their caregiver and emotional contagion thus, the automatic mimicry and synchronisation of emotional expressions plays a crucial role in co-regulation.

Through a Polyvagal Theory lens, it can be conceptualised that the root cause of self-defeating behaviours is a cumulative effect of many things, including life traumas. The child is not 'acting out' rather it is their nervous system's best attempt to survive.

Understanding that the vagus nerve serves as a neurophysiological map for the child to tell the story through their nervous system is important if we are to employ techniques to promote safety. Making therapeutic contact moment by moment, we "are engaging profound processes that tap into essential life forces in ourselves and in those we work with … Emotions are deepened in intensity and sustained in time when they are intersubjectively shared. This occurs at moments of deep contact" (Whitehead, 2006). Hence, the therapist's presence is vital in support of co-regulation and is the core of the work once *safety, safety, and safety* have been established.

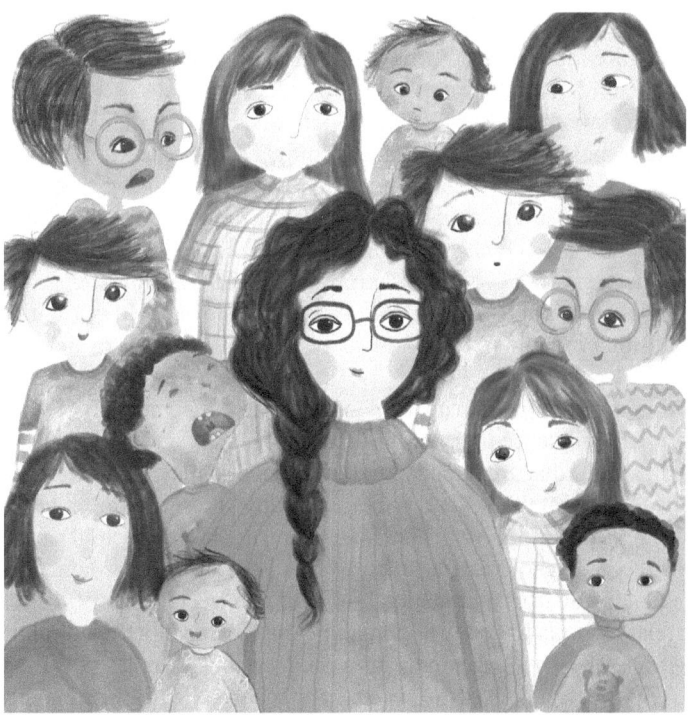

Figure 7.3 Therapist and her clients.

As therapists, we have likely trained in different modalities, all of which are valid. A Polyvagal framework can be integrated into any modality or therapeutic approach, as the autonomic nervous system does not discriminate. The goal is to strengthen the client's capacity to 'return home' and access the vagally mediated position of homeostasis. We need to be authentic in our interactions and transparent with our own mental processes as staying present in the here-and-now supports the child to feel safe. Badenoch (2018b) describes this external regulation from the therapist as the 'ventral embrace' suggesting that when a child's window of tolerance meets and joins up with the therapist's window of tolerance, the child can explore sympathetic arousal whist being regulated by the therapist. Fundamentally, when the child feels safe, their nervous system transitions to the AWAKE State often meaning that therapy is more impactful.

Alongside Carl Rogers' three core conditions of empathy, unconditional positive regard, and genuineness we also want to hold the position of curiosity, predictability, and familiarity. Being curious about what is happening in the child's nervous system is important as it helps us to conceptualise and recognise that their behaviours are their nervous system's best attempt to survive. Maroda (2004) challenges therapists to ponder an essential clinical problem: "How do you relate empathically to an unexpressed emotion?".

We have already considered how our client's autonomic nervous system's state can be understood through physiological markers. A smiling face and steady voice convey reassurance and openness, while a blank expression signals defensiveness and unease. Maintaining eye contact and engaging with speech become difficult when in the ALARM State with a racing heart. In the AVOID State, decreased heart rate limits facial movement and vocal melody. Children in the AWAKE State exhibit expressive, receptive behaviour, with a strong connection between facial expressions and emotions, characterised by natural vocal intonation, rhythmic speech, and smiles. How a child engages in play and therapeutic activities is also a strong indicator of nervous system activation.

A child therapist must remain vigilant to a client's perception of threat as this will profoundly influence their receptiveness to therapy and engagement in activities. Any activities that are intended to be therapeutic may inadvertently trigger or exacerbate feelings of fear and need to be carefully tailored to the child's emotional state and level of comfort. By understanding and addressing a child's perception of threat, the therapist can create a supportive and nurturing environment conducive to healing and growth. Additionally, by being attuned to signs of distress or discomfort related to perceived threats, the therapist can adapt interventions in real-time to ensure the child remains within their optimal window of tolerance. The *State of Play Reference List*© below summarises the client's potential play capacity and related physiological markers to help therapists identify where their client might be oriented:

State of Play Reference List©

ANS 'A' state	Polyvagal lens	Client presentation	
AWAKE State	• Social engagement • Seeking connection • Reciprocal cues of Safety and Trust • Homeostasis • Optimal zone of arousal	Play Capacity	• Receptive to the therapeutic relationship • Desire to engage with the self, therapist, and environment • Curious • Creative • Playful • Collaborative play • Blending of States of arousal • Co-regulation of each other's physiological states
		Physiological Markers	• Speaks rhythmically • Speaks with appropriate volume • Responds to your voice • Follows instructions • Appropriate affect • Spontaneity in the upper part of the face • Makes eye contact • Offers face-to-face gaze • Reactive pupils
ALARM State	• Mobilisation • Perceived threat • Flight • Flight • Freeze • Hyper-aroused	Play Capacity	• Compulsive repetition • Lack of catharsis • Messy and chaotic • Moving around • Putting things in their mouth • Body can't keep still • Hypervigilent • Lack of playfulness • Wanting to go to the toilet • Meltdowns • Tantrums • Agitated or aggressive • Poor sleep • Digestion problems • Obsessive-compulsive behaviour
		Physiological Markers	• Unable to read or respond to your vocal prosody • Unable to follow instructions • Reactive to ambient noise • Speaks with inappropriate volume • Dilated pupils • Frequent visits to the toilet

AVOID State	• Immobilisation	Play Capacity	• Little interest in the therapeutic alliance
	• Conserving energy		• Independent
	• Perceived threat is overwhelming		• Plays on their own
			• Turning away
			• Little communication
	• Hypo-aroused		• Quietly observes
	• Shutdown		• Does not actively participate
			• Dissociated/Frozen
			• Signs of depression
			• Disconnected
			• Lethargic
			• Difficulty articulating thoughts
		Physiological Markers	• Fixed gaze
			• Unable to sustain eye contact
			• Unable to offer face-to-face gaze
			• Speaks in a monotone voice
			• Flat facial affect
			• Constricted pupils
			• Unable to follow instructions

Once the relational safety is established then more directive approaches, techniques, and activities can be used to stretch the client's window of tolerance. Bromberg (2006) also points out that the therapeutic relationship must "feel safe but not perfectly safe … as there would be no potential for safe surprises". The goal of therapy through the Polyvagal lens is often for the child to have the flexibility to move in and out of ANS 'A' States of defence back to connectedness. Therapist awareness of breathing, mirroring facial expressions, matching vocal tone, offering visualisation, and comfort objects all support nervous system regulation. In addition, we can incorporate the use of the creative tool kit and offer a range of rhythmic activities and expressive movement activities to children including, holding a fidget toy, drinking through a straw, singing, humming, drawing, playing hide and seek, bubbles, and creating a ritual. These activities alongside many others, help the child strengthen their vagal brake and facilitate integration of the ANS.

When Emma first accessed therapy, she was rigid in the way that she played and in her use of the creative toolkit. She did not want to engage with the therapist, preferring to play on her own. Emma was in the AVOID State. The therapist noticed that Emma liked to go over to the 'fidget box' and would choose a toy that she could hold in one hand whilst drawing, using the sand, or playing with the dolls. Emma had moved into the ALARM State. Being aware of proximity in relation to Emma, the therapist would pick up a fidget toy, gently squeeze it in her hand and using a calm voice observe, track, and reflect some of Emma's movements and play. Gradually, Emma became more curious about the fidget toy that the therapist was holding and together, they would hide and find the fidget toys. Emma was in her AWAKE State, connected and engaged with the therapist, with the toys and within the therapy room.

The Super Protector©

Communicating and telling the story of the nervous system to help client understanding may include 'Your Body: The Super Protector©'. A creative psycho-education tool, it is designed to assist therapists in explaining to clients how the body responds involuntarily to safety and danger. Two versions of this illustrated guide are available, one for children and one for young people. Each provides professionals with clear, step-by-step instructions, utilising creative activities and strategies to help clients become familiar with the workings of their nervous system and how to read bodily signals when moving into protective responses. Reviewed by Stephen Porges and described by Lisa Dion as "a great educational tool, a must have for all Play Therapists", The Super Protector© helps the client to understand their body's reactions without conscious awareness removing a sense of shame around involuntary autonomic behaviours.

It is highly likely that Ezra has an oversensitive 'smoke alarm' and mismatched neuroception due to his early life trauma and the subsequent medical interventions and surgeries that he has received which, will be ongoing. When setting up the therapy room, the therapist chose to leave 'Your Body: The Super Protector' near the therapeutic story books. After a few sessions, Ezra became interested and started to ask questions about it. Over several sessions, the therapist titrated information to Ezra and when it was felt appropriate, sat with him explaining about his ANS and connecting it to the illustrated guide. Ezra asked many questions. The therapist was able to connect his burn injury trauma, hospital stays and behaviours to his ANS and ANS 'A' States. The age-appropriate graphics and supporting text gave Ezra a language to help him to understand his body.

Parental Engagement

The role of the therapist is to consider the clinical landscape and decide whether to work individually with the child or dyadically with the parent-child. Parental engagement is important to provide context and information and for the therapist to gain a sense of the parents' struggles/concerns.

When first meeting the parent and in subsequent appointments, sometimes we notice that the parents' capacity to represent, give meaning, and reflect the child's mind is not supported by their ability to be a co-organiser and co-regulator. It would always be our intention to create and offer a welcoming environment to the caregiver. We are open to holding their distress and hearing their experiences. We accept that their ANS will be scanning for cues of safety and cues of danger, therefore we need to be prepared for different reactions. Just as we do for our clients, we are listening and noticing the parents' embodied responses. Showing kindness and compassion for them and their child, we co-regulate by being a soothing presence helping the caregiver to stay with their here-and-now feelings as they are held, valued, and understood by us.

Through the referral process we are always thinking about what the most appropriate and conducive therapeutic intervention might be. Both the attachment theory and the Polyvagal Theory consider that the co-regulating relationship between the primary caregiver and child is of critical importance and the most effective way of mitigating psychological distress. As such, dyadic work may be the most beneficial approach. Through offering a playful "holding environment" (Winnicott, 1953) for both the parent and the child, the therapist empowers the parent to offer the core conditions to their child.

The Polyvagal Theory offers therapists valuable insight into the physiological underpinning of the parent-child relationship. For those therapists trained to offer parent-child dyadic interventions, part of the work is to enable the parent to identify and address difficulties within the relationship with their child. When Polyvagal principles are incorporated, the therapist can help the parent to recognise and respond to the child's ANS 'A' States. Guiding them to understand when their child has moved into the ALARM State or AVOID State will help in their understanding of why certain behaviours are emerging. Through a Polyvagal lens, we can support the parent to be more attuned and responsive in their caregiving behaviours. This leads to the development of co-regulation, wherein the parent will experience the child moving into the AWAKE State.

Amira's parents, Leyla and Ali have agreed to access a parent-child dyadic intervention. The therapist begins by offering four parent consultation sessions with them to gain an understanding of how they experience Amira and their mentalisation capacities. Titrating information about the Polyvagal Theory, the therapist uses The Super Protector© to help them to understand the ANS 'A' States connecting Amira's behaviours to how her body is showing distress. The therapist also talks about hierarchy. Presenting the AWAKE, ALARM and AVOID States, the therapist links this to neuroception and vagal tone as Amira is often under stress and her sense of neuroception leans towards cues of danger. In addition, Amira's vagal tone is underdeveloped because there have been minimal opportunities provided by Layla or Ali to support her with this. The therapist uses aspects of the creative tool kit to demonstrate the Polyvagal Theory including sand objects, dolls, puppets.

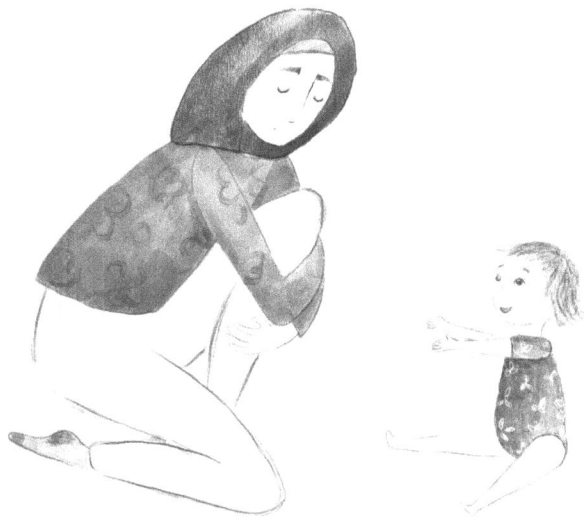

Figure 7.4 Leyla and Amira.

There are a range of interventions that support the parent-child dyad, including Theraplay®, Circle of Security®, Dyadic Developmental Psychotherapy, Video Interaction Guidance, and Filial Therapy. All of these approaches focus on strengthening the parent's capacity to engage with their child and reflexively respond to the child's ANS 'A' States in the present. In dyadic work, the child retains the position of 'client', however, this intersubjective process will be impactful for the parent. Oftentimes, parents we work with have experienced missed opportunities in early childhood themselves. The therapist's benign and caring presence can illicit strong feelings in the parent which will need to be attended to and looked after in order for them to be able to do this for their child.

If we observe that the parent has a mismatched autonomic nervous system and is struggling to be emotionally available and responsive to their child's needs, it may not be beneficial for them to partake in their child's therapy session. We know that the ANS can mirror another nervous system through emotional contagion, where individuals automatically mimic and synchronise their emotional states with those of others. From an autonomic perspective, we may conceptualise that there is a high probability that a parent who shows signs of stress and anxiety will be a mirror to their child, leading to them having a shared experience of embodied and autonomic emotional arousal. Through the lens of the Polyvagal Theory, this can be highly damaging for the child's ANS as the body scans for cues of danger rather than cues of safety.

Symbolic Repair©

Symbolic Repair© is a model for reparation in therapy. It in the context of the Polyvagal Theory, it can support the child's ANS to be vagally mediated through modelling attachment principles in the experience of co-regulation. As the therapist remains alongside, witnessing, and supporting the child, metaphorical and play processes within the therapist-child dyad symbolic repair© can "act as a vehicle for change" (Russ, 2004). If the therapist remains in the AWAKE State, we see that their calm and regulated autonomic state can help soothe and regulate the child leading to a shared state of physiological calmness. In these moments, the child's nervous system has responded to the therapist's nervous system, they have become synchronised in the AWAKE State. From a polyvagal and neurobiological perspective, "if the child can have an embodied experience of physiological synchrony, the wisdom of neurobiology will support right brain to right brain activity holding the possibility for the child to attach through the healing qualities of metaphor and imaginative play within the therapeutic dyad" (O'Neill, 2023).

Although decisions made by the therapist are contextual in guiding responses to the child, we continue to 'hold' the parent in mind, honouring the bravery of both them and their child.

Teddy has a fractured relationship with his mum, Jemma. He lives with his elderly grandparents, Betty, and Charles under a Special Guardianship Order. There are concerns about who will care for Teddy when they are no longer able to. It is hoped that in the future there will be a therapeutic intervention to support reunification between Teddy and Jemma. Currently, it would not be appropriate for the therapist to offer parent-child therapy as Jemma is not able to mentalise Teddy or offer co-regulation. The therapist made a clinical decision to offer Teddy non-directive play therapy. They recognised that their presence and the creative toolkit afforded the possibility that the therapeutic relationship could simulate the experience of nurture in infancy through metaphor and imaginative play. The intended outcome was that symbolic repair© would facilitate reparative processes that Teddy missed as an infant before living with Betty and Charles. This would support the regulation of Teddy's stress response system and the strengthening of his vagal brake.

According to Ana Gomez, as therapists we need to be able to 'zoom in and zoom' out of self and others. At any given point we must have an awareness of the embodied mind of the child and notice what is emerging for us. Moment to moment decision-making requires the therapist to be aware and conscious as this is the nucleus of any psychotherapeutic process. Alongside this, we remain alert to the emergence of regression in the child's presentation. Within the therapeutic process, children will revisit developmental stages and revisit and revisit, until their innate wisdom to repair has been satisfied. The child's capacity to move on from an earlier unmet need is dependent on the therapist's attendance to that need. When core conditions are experienced, the client is free to gently explore the next wound. In the context of the Polyvagal Theory, we can compare different processes within child-centred therapy.

Processes in Child-Centred Therapy through a Polyvagal Lens©

Therapeutic process	Polyvagal process	Child-centred response
Feel Safe	Neuroception of safety	• Accept the child for who they are • Sending cues of safety • Therapist actively self-regulates
Awareness of feelings	Exercise neural brake	• Tracking clients' actions • Therapist reflects on their own States • Keeping client within their Window of Tolerance
Dance of attachment	Co-regulation	• Use of 'we' statements • Bodily Reflections • Moving with regression
Express feelings	Development of social engagement system	• Reflect client's States and emotions • Development of Interoception
Development of resilience	Neural expectancies of safety	• Therapist tracks and expands client's exploration through verbal responses or activities • Therapist is curious about the client's real-life

The therapist's presence is vital as we communicate a steady stream of 'play signals' which helps the child to remain within the safety of their autonomic window of tolerance. Furthermore, play allows the child to apply their vagal brake by pretending without real threat or danger and, being connected but at the same time tolerating distress. This process encourages co-regulation which will result in the client being able to manage their big feelings in a more appropriate way.

> *Tom likes to play sword fights. He puts the therapist and himself in the role of pirates and gives instructions as to how they should play. As Tom and the therapist play, he is mobilised and in heightened arousal. The play is active, and Tom is in his ALARM State. As they continue, Tom is practicing utilising his vagal brake. There is a blending of the parasympathetic and the sympathetic without triggering protective responses. Although Tom becomes mobilised, he is in social play. There is no threat or danger to Tom's ANS as he is connected and engaging playfully with the therapist. Tom is in his AWAKE State.*

Returning to the creative toolkit and as previously discussed in Chapter 6, play and metaphorical processes allow for hybrid autonomic states which can address something that is really big with something that can be creative and fun. At the core of the work is the offering of familiarity and predictability that supports autonomic homeostasis for the client. If we can intervene early, it can change the child's trajectory as little micro moments can make a difference which can have a lifelong impact on the autonomic nervous system.

Chapter 8

Scaffolding Caregivers and Teachers

The ideal interpersonal trajectory starts with the infant's total dependency on a key adult, leading to interdependency through relationships with multiple adults, resulting (eventually) in independence and self-regulation. In the preceding chapters, we have discussed the vulnerability of the newborn infant as it leaves the safety of the womb and its innate drive to secure external support to manage its autonomic regulation. This biological motivation for emotions to be regulated interpersonally by a safe adult is the necessary first step in developing self-regulation. The human capacity to self-regulate evolves over time and the amount of co-regulatory input needed will vary throughout different life stages. Rosanbalm and Murray (2017) invite us to consider that children and young people have the capacity to fill their own self-regulation "bucket" at varying levels, depending on their developmental stage and lived experience. But to successfully manage their emotions and behaviours they will always need an adult to fill the remainder of their "bucket" through co-regulation. Regardless of the age or stage of the child, they will need dependable adults to offer them a felt sense of safety and a predictable environment.

A child who is accessing weekly therapy will typically spend less than an hour a week with their therapist. Thirty-two hours per week are spent in school and the remainder of the time (around eighty waking hours) will be spent with caregivers. Parents provide the immediate and most influential environment for children, with teachers and schools coming a very close second. Indeed, a study by the Centre for Economic Performance demonstrates that the teacher's influence on the mental health of students is as significant as their influence on academic results. Involving parents in the therapeutic process indubitably offers more favourable outcomes for our clients. Working alongside teachers has the potential for positive consequences for all children under their care.

This chapter encourages you to share theoretical concepts with the most influential adults in the client's life. Through a polyvagal framework, parents and teachers can be helped to better understand and respond to the neurobiological underpinnings of stress and engagement in the home and the classroom. We will start by thinking about your first meeting, and offering additions to your typical intake process. Your psychoeducation toolkit will be broadened to include activities that will make

DOI: 10.4324/9781003412571-9

the organising principles of the Polyvagal Theory accessible and applicable. The needs and capacities of parents and teachers will be considered. Some may benefit from a cognitive and intellectual approach, wherein a scientific foundation of neurobiology supports them to better understand the child. For others, a greater advantage will be made through embodied non-verbal communication. Supporting them to experience reciprocity you will encourage their mirror neurons to 'get busy' and have a felt sense of attunement and positive regard. Finally, we will journey through review meetings and endings, looking at each stage through a polyvagal lens.

First Meeting with Parents

Lisa Dion once noted "No parent ever gives birth and thinks, 'I can't wait to meet my child's therapist'". Whatever the reason you are having a first meeting with a parent, it is highly likely they are living with challenge and upset. Whether that parent is familiar and comfortable with the therapeutic process or is new to it, seeking therapeutic support for their child indicates that somewhere their wishes and dreams have gone awry. They may perceive that they are not coping or doing a good enough job as a parent without your help.

In the majority of cases, prior to an initial meeting, a referral will have been made indicating a general area of need and reason why therapeutic intervention is being sought. From this moment, the therapist will consciously (intellectually) and unconsciously (physiologically) respond to the data given. Our theoretical 'mind-library' will search for relevant frameworks and concepts. Our personal histories will find ways to relate or reject. We will experience a visceral response to the information shared and assumptions about the child and parents will be made. We simply can't help it.

Whilst the overarching reason for meeting a parent is for the therapist to garner information about the child's history and difficulties, this first meeting also lays the foundation for you to connect and co-regulate with the parent. With some parents, this is a seamless process. We find commonality and have a natural flow of empathy which allows us to remain in the AWAKE State and offer a persistent neuroception of safety. But what of those parents who have a seeming disregard for therapeutic intervention? Or those about whom we have a level of judgement, prejudice, or even trepidation?

It would be entirely dishonest to pretend that we are open and unbiased in all parental interactions. The way some parents might behave towards us or speak about their children can cause even the most masterful therapist to feel enraged or despairing. We need to remember that parents will be bringing their own history and experiences of being with a professional which may not have been positive. They may have been repeatedly called into school or involved with social services and other professionals. They may have their own unresolved childhood wounds, unlikely to be socially engaged or ready to connect.

As ever, we must first attend to ourselves, pay attention to our autonomic states, and orient ourselves to a safe and social position. Without doing so, it is highly likely that we will be pulled into joining the parent's chaos, fear, or disconnection. We may project these back into the family system. As intentional professionals, we have the capacity to understand the parent's State. By reading their facial expressions, listening to their tone of voice, noticing their posture and gestures we can consider how this makes us feel. It is only when we have a calm physiological State of our own, that we can send cues of safety, which will in turn engender social connectedness. This is all essential if we want to get a productive and meaningful intake meeting underway with a stabilised parent who has the capacity to work alongside you.

Taking this into account, you may consider whether the typical model of a one-off intake meeting is suitable for a parent who has not yet navigated a physiological sense of safety. Some parents may need multiple interactions with you to build the capacity for trust and collaboration.

Emma had been referred to therapy by her school and whilst her mother Dawn gave consent, she was reluctant to take part in face-to-face meetings, citing childcare difficulties as her main issue. It was agreed that the first meeting would take place online. Dawn eventually arrived onscreen 10 minutes late, flustered, irritated, and stressed.

Dawn repeatedly got up and down from her chair. Her body needed to move, her breath was fast, and she avoided eye contact through the computer screen.

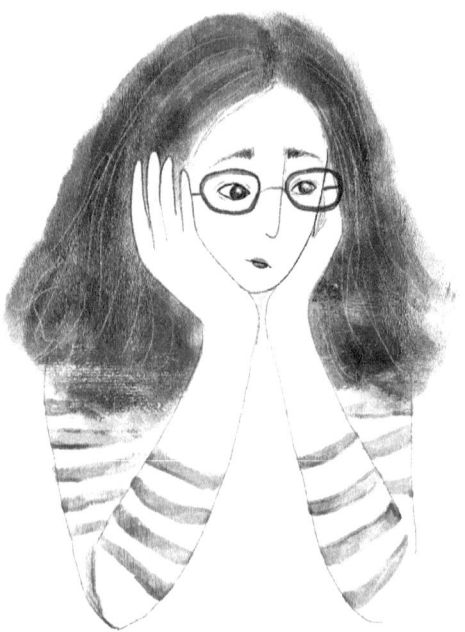

Figure 8.1 Dawn.

Any attempt to begin a formalised intake process would have been over-whelming for Dawn and would not have elicited connection. She was in the ALARM State and unable to detect cues of safety or think rationally. Her nervous system required the therapist to utilise their social engagement system (tone of voice and facial expression), recruit their mirror neurons (use of breath, stretching, leaning into their chair) to give meaning to Dawn's experience.

Dawn was wary of external support, having felt judged by both social services and her older children's school. When therapy for Emma was recommend to Dawn, she expressed surprise and indifference to the process. It was apparent that Dawn did not view this meeting as an opportunity to get support, rather it was a hoop to jump so "meddling do-gooders would leave me alone" (as she shared in a later meeting!!). She needed to be seen, heard and related to. Her older two children were at times frightening, aggressive, protecting themselves through mobilization. Whereas Emma defended herself by shutting down and disappearing. Dawn seemed to oscillate between the two positions. She relied on her relationship with her partner Helen for fleeting moments of connection in a world that felt overwhelming, chaotic and rejecting.

The intake process took place over three appointments. The first two meetings were gentle and slow, providing Dawn with an opportunity to share her own experiences and be listened to. For the third meeting, Dawn opted for a face-to-face appointment wherein she openly shared details about Emma's behaviour and history.

We appreciate that not all work settings or budgets allow the opportunity to extend to multiple intake meetings with parents. It is important, however, for us to consider the level of expectation we might be placing on them. This might result in information being distorted or prevent parental engagement from developing. Whilst there is a strong clinical basis for getting as much information as possible about the client's background and life circumstances, prioritising relationship building will, in the long run, be a more productive outcome. Data gathering can come later.

First Meeting with Teachers

Broadly speaking, education systems are designed to teach children who can learn. Demands and expectations are high. Schools are product-driven environments where students and staff are measured and assessed according to generalised competency matrices.

Daily, teachers engage with pupils, parents, colleagues, and administrators carrying out a multitude of tasks. We estimate that the average teacher could be communicating with up to sixty other nervous systems in one day. In the classroom, the nervous system of each student will be responding to moment-to-moment data. This will likely include multiple children who have mismatched 'Smoke Alarms', experiencing the world from an activated ALARM State or a shutdown AVOID State. Teachers will be attempting to disseminate learning to children who are stuck in their emotional brains. They may be responding to behaviours and reactions from students that probably have very little to do with the here and now. To learn, students need to be in a socially engaged position. To teach, teachers need to be in a socially engaged position. For a school system to function all parties must experience a neuroception of safety to access higher brain structures.

When meeting teachers, time is often limited and it can be tempting to dive in and offer psychoeducation, well-meaning ideas, or the implementation of new strategies. Before any of this, we need to listen to their experience and get an understanding of what it is like for them to teach our clients. Assuming you have had the opportunity to meet with your client and their parent, you will be holding two experiences of how they operate. In the home and in the therapy space. Often children will respond to a school environment in an altogether different way. It is important to get the teacher's expertise on how the child orients in an educational setting. In prioritising attentive listening, two outcomes are achieved. Firstly, we are given a golden opportunity to get a big-picture view of how our client's interactions change or remain rigid according to the setting or circumstances they are navigating. Secondly, we can show genuine interest in the teacher's experiences and challenges, fostering a sense of collaboration and shared investment in the child's wellbeing.

Utilising the Polyvagal Framework for Case Conceptualisation

The principles of the Polyvagal Theory can be utilised by therapists as part of their formal intake procedure to consider a client's physiological response to the world in which they live. We have designed the Child Social Engagement Capacity Questionnaire© (CSECQ) to support therapists in beginning the process of formulating an understanding of their client's autonomic responses to the environment. This assists the therapist with Case Conceptualisation in the context of three important concepts: 1) Goal Setting, 2) Adult Mentalisation, and 3) Psychoeducational Needs

The first section, *Perception of Threat*, has 10 questions and is divided into four categories: Novel Events, Autonomic States, Pathways to Safety, and Triggers. The second section, *Orienting to Safety*, has six questions and two categories: Seeking Connection and Environmental Cues of Safety. It considers if the child has the capacity for Social Engagement and how this is achieved (Figures 8.2 and 8.3).

CSECQ

Child Social Engagement Capacity Questionnaire

	Section One: Perception of Threat	TICK IF A CONCERN	
1	Does the child like going to new places?		*Novel Events*
2	Does the child react to any changes in their routine or environment?		
3	When upset, distressed, or angry can the child listen to instructions?		*Autonomic States*
4	What kind of behaviour does the child engage in when they are upset, angry, or distressed?		
5	Does the child always respond in the same way if upset, angry, or distressed?		
6	Does the child ever seem distant or shutdown with adults or other children?		
7	What does the child need to calm down?		*Pathway to safety*
8	How long does it take for the child to calm down after they are distressed?		
9	Are there any particular people, places, sounds, or events that cause the child to feel upset, angry, or distressed?		*Trigger*
10	Do the child's behaviours make sense to you?		

Figure 8.2 Child Social Engagement Capacity Questionnaire© (CSECQ).

CSECQ

Child Social Engagement Capacity Questionnaire

	Section Two: Orienting to Safety	TICK IF A CONCERN	
11	Who is the child closest to?		*Seeking Connection*
12	How does the child demonstrate their closeness (proximity, touch, behaviours)?		
13	How does the child seek out comfort from others?		
14	Is there a place that seems to make the child feel most relaxed or happy?		*Environmental Cues of Safety*
15	When and where is the child able to remain socially engaged (e.g. play, relax, join in conversations, follow instructions)?		
16	Is there a game, activity, or type of play that the child particularly enjoys?		

Figure 8.3

Goal Setting

The polyvagal framework provides therapists with a unique set of goals that can measure the child's regulatory capacity. The following are suggested goals that the therapist can hold in mind when considering the efficacy of their work:

- Can the child return to Ventral Vagal (Safe and Social) State?
- Does the child have an awareness of which state they are in?

- Is the child able to adaptively move movement between autonomic states?
- Has the child got high Vagal Tone?
- Is there an established Ventral Brake?

The CSECQ obtains information about the adult's perception of the child's autonomic states and how well they are able to orient themselves to a felt sense of safety. Below is a summary of the purpose of the questions in each category:

Perception of threat

Q1-2	These questions explore how the child's system can cope with change. Children and young people who do not perceive that they have a path to safety will not risk novel experiences. This can indicate low vagal tone as the child is unable to move into unpredictable situations without becoming activated and their vagal brake is unable to distinguish real threat from perceived threat.	*Novel Events*
Q3-6	These questions consider the child's physiological response to upset, distress, or anger. Answers to these questions can indicate whether the child has a bias towards mobilisation, immobilisation, or both; as well as indicating whether the child has an established vagal brake.	*Autonomic States*
Q7-8	These questions consider the child's capacity for a ventral vagal position. Answers to these questions may inform you as to whether the dysregulated child relies on adapted self-soothing patterns or calls on the nervous system of a trusted adult.	*Pathway to safety*
Q9-10	Enquiring about triggers helps reveal whether the child's behaviours are matched or mismatched. If the parent is unable to make sense of the behaviour, or dysregulation seems to occur compulsively, it could indicate that the child is living in a protective position and unable to discern threats from safety.	*Trigger*

Section 2, Orienting to Safety, is relevant to the relational goals of therapy. This section of the CSECQ is interested in how the child uses their social engagement system and whether they can find safety in the environment. Asking about the child's preferred types of play and how they play will help you think about their capacity to blend their Social Engagement System with sympathetic activation. A child who can engage in connected intimacy is demonstrating they can blend their Dorsal and Social Engagement Systems. The information garnered from Section Two is critical for the therapist to consider whether their benign and caring presence may trigger The Needs Paradox® and generate feelings of fear and threat or be a source of safety for the child.

Orienting to safety

Q11-12	These questions explore whether the child's social engagement system is activated, and it detects cues of safety through neuroception. Answers to these questions will indicate whether the child uses the relationship as a tool to co-regulate their effect, behaviours, and physiological state.	*Seeking Connection*
Q13-15	These final questions ask whether there are certain environmental or sensorial conditions that offer a neuroception of safety. The therapist can use this information to consider whether the therapeutic environment they are offering is conducive to the child's needs.	*Environmental Cues of Safety*

Listening to Dawn describe Emma's capacity for connection was difficult. Dawn noted that Emma was closest to her younger stepsiblings, seemed happiest playing with them in their bedroom together and very rarely sought proximity or comfort from the adults in her life. Dawn joked how Emma played babyish games with the younger children's toys. She never wanted to sit with the whole family and would be the first to clear up after a meal and then disappear upstairs.

Dawn's description of Emma signifies that she would likely find the intensity of the 1:1 therapeutic dyad challenging. She has organised herself not to rely on adults, preferring to be the caretaker and appeaser. It could not be assumed that Emma would be able to experience the therapeutic process as safe. It was important to consider ways to titrate Emma into receiving co-regulation and attunement. The CSECQ suggested that the primary therapeutic goal for Emma was to support her to be able to tolerate and utilise the therapist's social engagement system. This could support her to develop her own capacity for sympathetic-vagal balance.

Adult Mentalisation

Each question in the CSECQ requires the adult to step into the experience of the child and consider the world from their perspective. This invites the adult to consider how they experience and understand their relationship with the child and how they feel about the child's behaviour. Mentalisation refers to the adult's capacity to understand the internal experiences of the child and see the connection between the child's emotions and their actions. An adult with a mentalising capacity can hold the child's mental state in mind and understand that behaviours result from the child's inner experiences and feelings.

> *When Hannah's mother Claire was asked "What does Hannah need to calm down?", she answered, "Hannah needs to know I am there, but she normally doesn't like it if I hug her when she isn't ready. I sit next to her and tell her I am sorry that she is feeling sad and that I am ready for a cuddle whenever she needs one. She needs me to be quiet with her most of the time."*

Claire's response indicates that she is aware that Hannah's upset belongs to her. She doesn't become enmeshed with Hannah's feelings and mentalises about Hannah's internal state of *sad*. Claire can separate herself from Hannah's pain and understands that Hannah will be able to use her as a tool of comfort and regulation when she needs it. In using the descriptors *normally* and *most of the time*, Claire is indicating that she understands that Hannah has various emotions and internal states that can require different responses from her. Claire is not certain about Hannah's needs which is a crucial aspect of mentalisation. Parents are not mind readers after all and can only guess what their children are feeling and needing. It is due to Claire's mentalising capacity that she referred Hannah to therapy as she understood that her own mental states were vulnerable due to the loss of her mother, resulting in a compromised capacity to hold her daughter's grief.

> *Tom's mother, Michelle, had a harder time trying to imagine what might be motivating his behaviours. When he is dysregulated, Tom rejects Michelle leaving her feeling confused and frustrated. There were frequent misunderstandings about Tom's needs and the cause of his meltdowns. He often seemed to misread Michelle's intentions when she attempted to provide comfort or parent him.*

> *When Michelle was asked "How does Tom seek out comfort from others?" Michelle responded: "He likes a cuddle, but only on his terms. If he's in a bad mood, don't even think of trying to hug him if he hasn't asked for it, he just hits you and its horrible. It's so hard because he always gets angry with me when I am doing something for him. Like cooking his dinner, I have to feed him, and he loves his food. I just don't know what he thinks I am supposed to do. It always ends in both of us crying and waiting for Paul to get home and calm things down. The worst part is he's always so upset afterwards, like he has no idea what happened either.".*

Here Michelle hasn't been able to describe how Tom seeks comfort when he is dysregulated. She lacks curiosity as to why he turns to activated behaviours, talking

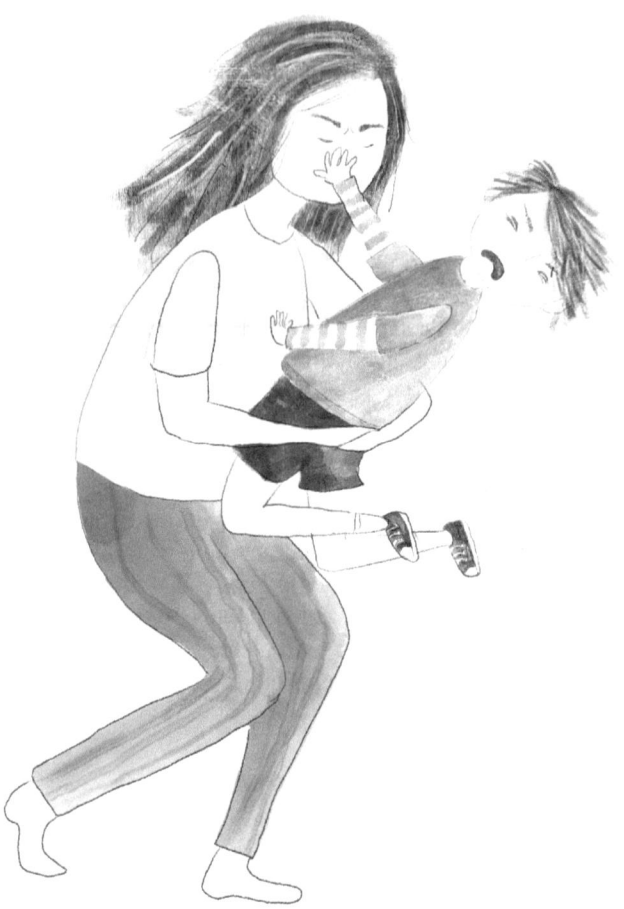

Figure 8.4 Tom and Michelle.

more about her experience and how he won't let her comfort him. She describes how Tom *"always gets angry"*, her perception is that he only has one internal state. She attributes his dysregulation to external factors *"doing something for him"*, not accounting for his internal experience when she leaves him. Michelle finds it very challenging not to become enmeshed in Tom's upset. She describes how she too is often left in tears with a sense of hopelessness, waiting for her husband to give her the support that she needs. Due to his early trauma, Tom can offer confusing signals that are very hard for his parents to read. Michelle has been utterly committed to creating a safe and loving home for Tom yet continues to feel rejected by him. Her capacity to regulate in the face of Tom's behaviours is limited and her own protective responses are triggered.

Psychoeducational Needs

Psychoeducation can be a pivotal aspect in helping parents and teachers gain relevant insight and help provide a supportive environment for the child. However, we must be sensitive to their capacity and openness to engaging in psychoeducation. We need to be alert to the level of demand we place on parents and teachers, reminding ourselves that any perceived resistance to new knowledge may come from a place of exhaustion or overwhelm, rather than lack of care or interest. Posing the specific questions suggested in the CSECQ allows the therapist to gauge the adult's understanding of the context of the child's behaviours. We are then able to carefully extend an offer to share our insights and perspectives through a polyvagal lens, regarding potential explanations for the child's behaviour.

Having confirmed a readiness to engage, a tailored package of appropriately targeted psychoeducation can be created which can have a marked impact on how an adult thinks about and responds to the child. If we can effectively explain concepts of the Polyvagal Theory, adults can understand that the child's actions are automatic and have been adapted in service of survival.

One of the biggest barriers for therapists wishing to teach Polyvagal Theory's organising principles is the scientific and somewhat prohibitive language used to describe it. In its essence, however, it is an incredibly intuitive construct. All humans react and all humans need connection. The three principles of the Polyvagal Theory can be explained in relatable ways that are meaningful to the adult's own experiences as well as helping them to understand the child's actions.

Neuroception

Introducing this concept by orienting the adult to a universal experience is a great tool. You could ask if they have ever met someone who they get a funny feeling about for no reason at all. This illustrates the autonomic threat response perfectly. Alternatively, you could talk about gut feelings, how your body tells you something is right or wrong long before your brain has made a decision about it. Whilst none of these are exactly scientific explainers, they do open the door for further discussion about why our bodies respond to data in the environment.

In Chapter 7, you were introduced to The Super Protector©. We would encourage you to recruit this tool to help adults understand the concepts of neuroception and hierarchy. Along with helping develop an understanding of the child's involuntary response to threat, this is a great opportunity to gently invite the adult to consider their own ANS 'A' States.

Using Animal Metaphors to Explain Hierarchy

Since all mammals share the same autonomic response to threat, it may be helpful to use examples of how animals respond as an engaging way of exploring hierarchical responses. A rabbit and a dog provide the perfect example. Set the scene by describing a rabbit in a field and ask the adult to imagine the rabbit hopping about in the sunshine. Next, ask them to imagine that the rabbit sees a dog in the corner of the field. It stands on its hind legs looking for other rabbits; at this point, the rabbit is in the AWAKE State. The dog sees the rabbit and starts running towards it. Immediately the rabbit runs away desperately trying to flee the scene. It has moved into the ALARM State.

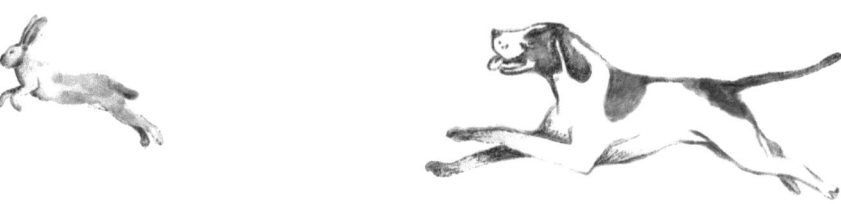

Figure 8.5 Dog chasing rabbit.

As the dog gets closer, the rabbit does its best to get away but is not quick enough. As soon as the dog catches it, the rabbit goes limp, collapses and its body hang in the dog's mouth. The rabbit is now in the AVOID State. The dog stops in its tracks. Confused it spits out the rabbit, sniffs at it, and wanders off. As soon as the dog has left the scene the rabbit jumps up and runs away. It is once again filled with energy and back into the ALARM State. Finally, the rabbit reaches the safety of its burrow. It returns to the AWAKE State.

This story explains the different hierarchical positions the body takes according to the perception of threat. Initially the rabbit remained in a socially engaged AWAKE State, seeking connection from other rabbits. As the threat increased the rabbit was mobilised to the ALARM State and needed to do something to protect itself. When the dog caught up with the rabbit mobilisation was no longer the optimal response. There was no option but to turn to the AVOID State, collapse and shutdown. Bidirectionally, the rabbit was able to return to the AWAKE State, having first mobilised away from the danger.

Animal Behaviour Game

Once the adult understands hierarchical responses to perceived threats, you can start to engender their curiosity about their own ANS 'A' States and those of the child. Using metaphor protects the adult as they can project their experience onto an animal. The Animal Behaviour Game encourages the adults to gain a clearer understanding of themselves without feeling exposed or judged.

This activity lends itself to multiple variations. You could use sand play miniatures, puppets, or clay/play doh figures. For the simple version, you need to prepare a piece of paper with eight different animals printed/drawn on it such as the diagram below.

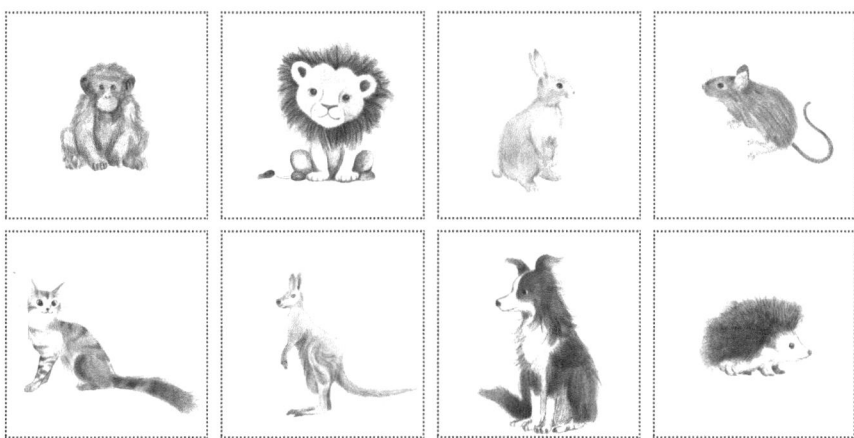

Figures 8.6–8.13 Animal behaviour game.

1 Start by asking the adult to think about how each animal responds to a threat. Help them organise these into ANS 'A' States (e.g., the hedgehog would move to the AVOID State. The lion and dog would move to the ALARM State).
2 Ask which animal the child most closely resembles when they are upset, distressed, or angry.
3 Explore whether the child responds the same way in all situations, or if events or people cause different autonomic responses.
4 Ask the adult to consider if they respond like any of these animals.
5 Consider whether the animal they have identified with can comfort the other animal.

The Animal Behaviour Game helped Michelle to identify the different autonomic states Tom would be triggered into when he perceived she was abandoning him. "He is like a kangaroo, boxing gloves on and in for the attack as soon as I need to do anything. This makes me become a hedgehog, I want to curl up into a ball." We talked about what a kangaroo might need when it is feeling defensive. Michelle identified that the kangaroo might need a calming animal that won't leave such as a koala bear. Through this process, Michelle understood that her dorsal response to Tom's anger was making him even more frightened and reactive. Tom had multiple experiences of abandonment in his early life and was primed to protect himself from it ever happening again.

The Animal Behaviour Game provides the perfect lead-in to introducing the final principal "Co-regulation".

Co-regulation

The teaching of co-regulation begins with us offering a warm, responsive, and supportive relationship to the adult we are working with. It is possible that parents and teachers we meet lacked an attuned caregiver themselves and have little experience of how these feels. We know that a dysregulated adult can lead to a dysregulated child and vice versa. In a school setting, it only takes one student in the ALARM State to become the class disruptor, transmitting their heightened responses to their peer group and leaving the teacher disarmed and overwhelmed. The teacher's emotional experience will shape the relationships they build with their students. In the same way a parent's affect and ability to connect has an impact on how their child perceives the world.

Co-regulation can only happen if the adult is in a regulated position themselves. Just as we need to be the emotional regulator for our clients, we need to offer the same conditions for the adults we are supporting so they can begin to appreciate the value of attending to themselves before attempting to support the child. Sharing the classic airline instruction: "Parents put your oxygen mask on first" applies beautifully here and supports adults to see the logic in looking after themselves to better look after the child. Flight attendants give this instruction as they know that an adult who leaves their oxygen mask last, will likely run out of air and be unable to help anyone else. The same applies to adults who don't attend to their own regulatory needs. They need to regulate themselves first, to have the capacity to help the child.

In order to co-regulate, the adult needs to respond flexibly to the challenges presented by their child, rather than reacting from a survival position. Using activities such as The Animal Behaviour Game invites adults to consider their bodily sensations in the face of the child's upset, distress, or anger. Since emotion regulation is dependent on awareness of sensory signals, it would be helpful to support adult to listen to their own body signals and be aware of what their body needs to return to a safe and social position. Stressed adults often minimise their own needs, feeling guilty if they take any time to centre themselves, but a barking dog is not going to offer a felt sense of safety to a frightened rabbit.

When you invite adults to listen to their sensory signals, you are familiarising them with interoception. Described as the 8th sensory system, interoception allows us to sense what is happening inside of our bodies. From a polyvagal perspective having interoceptive awareness is hugely important. It is the body's way of bringing neuroception to conscious awareness through identifying bodily sensations. Without interoception, we wouldn't understand any emotions at all. It is only when we become consciously aware of changes to our internal sensations that we can start to identify feelings such as excitement, happiness, and anger.

Adults often ask us to help the child express how they are feeling. Without a developed interoceptive awareness, this is impossible as the child has no conscious data on which to share their internal states. Interoceptive awareness can be hindered or blocked for a multitude of reasons including but not limited to trauma, depression, ASD, ADHD, and sensory processing challenges. Adults can be coached to help the child familiarise themselves with their internal States by providing a narrative for the child's changing States, alongside noticing their own.

Having identified Tom's perception of threat when he feels abandoned, the therapist supported his teacher to find ways to support his interoceptive awareness. The goal was to help Tom have a better understanding of the signals that his body gives him. Supporting Tom to develop interoceptive awareness was a three-stage process. To begin, his teacher was encouraged to share her internal States with Tom "My body feels heavy, it is telling me I am tired"; "My tummy has electricity in it, I am feeling excited". She then noticed out-loud the physiological changes in Tom, "Your hands are in tight fists, I wonder if you are feeling cross. Your jaw is clenched, I wonder if you are feeling frustrated." Finally, she was curious about how his body was feeling when she perceived a shift in his affect, "You seem worried about something, I wonder what your body is feeling. You threw your bag on the floor, is your tummy feeling jumbly?"

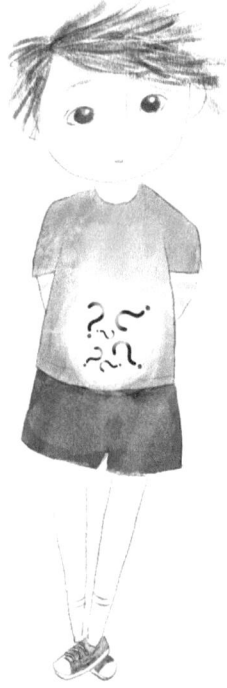

Figure 8.14 Interoception.

Offering adults the analogy of "put the crying baby down" is helpful for those who need a moment to recalibrate and attend to themselves. Anyone who has held a persistently crying baby understands that there are moments when the best thing to do is leave the baby in a safe place for a few moments. The adult can then gather themself before returning to another round of soothing. Adults with responsibility for hurt or challenged children may feel that they have no time or right to attend to their own needs. Unfortunately, the concept of self-care can become synonymous with self-centredness. In fact, self-care should be considered part of their duty of care. In the presence of a child's nervous system that is signalling danger and readiness to attack, it is essential for the adult to have access to self-regulation to meet the challenge.

To reconnect to self, it is helpful to identify the different resources that can help us to feel safe, connected, present and settled. In her book the *Polyvagal Theory in Therapy (2018)*, Deb Dana introduces us to the concept of glimmers, stressing the importance of identifying "accurate recognition of helpful …. experiences." Dana is careful to point out that that glimmers don't need to be substantial actions, instead they are "micro-moments that begin to shape our system in very gentle ways." Dana describes this as a process of anchoring to self. We have extended this metaphor and encourage therapist to help support adults to 'Identify their Safe Harbours' and become familiar with what they need to return to a regulated state.

Identifying Safe Harbours

A Safe Harbour offers a place that protects, repairs, and facilitates a safe ongoing journey. From a polyvagal perspective, we understand that our autonomic nervous system evaluates threat or safety within the environment, by listening to our bodies or in the presence of another nervous system. 'Identifying Safe Harbours' prompts a conversation about the available resources the adult you are supporting can utilise to return to a state of social engagement.

Who?

Consideration of the "Who" aspect involves helping the adult recognise supportive individuals that bring with them a connected AWAKE State that can be borrowed and co-regulated with. Help the adult identify the people in their lives that return to a Safe Harbour by making them feel seen. Who listens to them, laughs with them and validates their experience? Be curious about how often the adult links their nervous system to their people of safety.

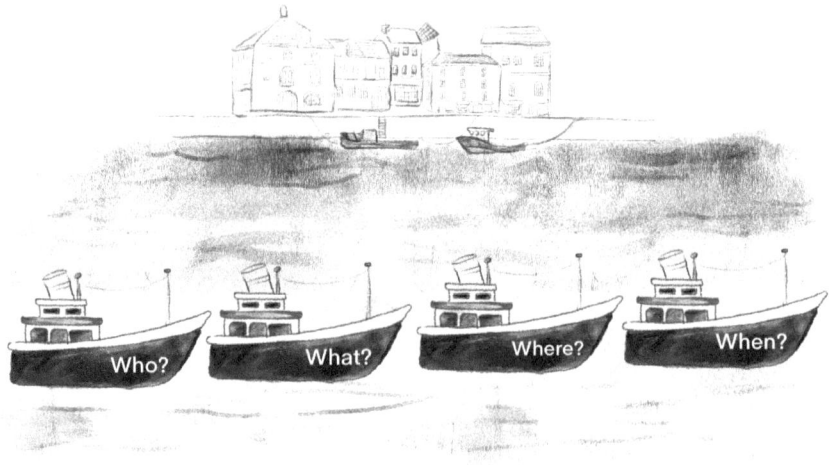

Figure 8.15 Safe Harbour.

What?

Through exploring the "What", the adult is supported to think about how they engage in self-regulation activities. You may help this process by inviting them to think about the times they feel most ok and ask them what their body is doing. Are they moving? Having moments of stillness? What is their breathing like? Do they sing or hum or dance? Finish by helping them to consider whether these activities can be adapted and implemented in a scaled-down manner and applied within their day. A quick 10-minute brisk walk can boost our mental alertness, energy levels, and overall positive mood (Mental Health Foundation, 2023).

Where?

The "Where" dimension will enhance awareness of the environment's positive aspects. Is there somewhere in the home which feels like a safe and calming space for the parent? A teacher might be supported to take a mental tour of the school, naming physical places that bring cues of safety. Do they need to take a moment outside in the fresh air? If this isn't possible, opening a window and taking a deep breath may be helpful.

When?

Addressing the "When" aspect involves a thoughtful exploration of the adult's busy schedule and well-being priorities. A compelling analogy compares prioritizing well-being to the decision of driving at 70 miles per hour instead of 80. While the faster speed saves a mere 6 seconds per mile, it significantly inflates fuel costs, exacerbates environmental impact, and heightens the risk of a road traffic accident. Initiating a conversation about the genuine value of prioritizing themselves, even for a moment, allows space for them to find a Safe Harbour for themselves in the present. In the slowing down, they will have the capacity to be emotionally available to the child in their care.

When adults are assisted in becoming aware of their own needs, they can acquire the skills to adjust their reactions. This enhances their ability to self-regulate and re-establish equilibrium, connecting with the AWAKE State. From this position, they will be communicating signals of safety to the child, able to read non-verbal cues and determine the child's neural capacity to take on demands.

ANS 'A' States and Learning

Without a felt sense of safety, children can't learn. In the home or classroom, adults may misinterpret the child's protective behaviours. A hyper-aroused child may shout out, fidget, move around, crash, bang, or annoy others. They may be labelled as oppositional or defiant when in the ALARM State. A hypo-aroused child may not answer, slump in their chair, refuse, or withdraw. They run the very real risk of being ignored or missed when they are in the AVOID State. Whatever behaviours the child is communicating, they are doing so in an attempt to regulate but are finding themselves stuck in a pattern of dysregulation. Once teachers and parents are alert to the different protective positions a child might have taken, we can help them to consider the related functional capacity to learn, complete tasks, and do what is asked of them.

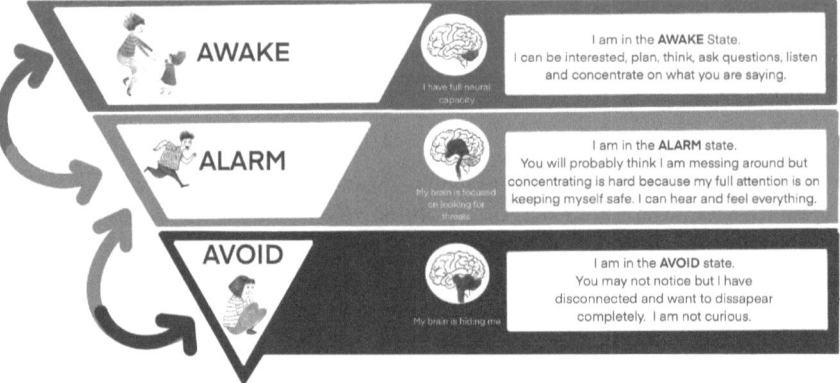

Figure 8.16 ANS 'A' States and learning.

Figure 8.16 demonstrates how optimal learning occurs when we engage the higher regions of our brain. If we find ourselves in the lower regions, our processing capabilities shift, leading to unsuccessful learning experiences.

The capacity to think and make choices is entirely dependent on the child having access to all brain regions. Acquiring knowledge includes the processes of encoding, consolidation, and retrieval, wherein the prefrontal cortex, hippocampus, and amygdala play pivotal roles. It is for this reason traditional behavioural approaches won't be successful for the dysregulated child. Reward charts, stickers, time out, or threatening to contact a more powerful adult such as another parent or headteacher are typical strategies employed in homes and schools. These approaches are very successful short-term strategies for well-adjusted and securely attached children with the capacity for self-regulation. They do not work for children who have experienced developmental trauma or have attachment strategies borne out of insecurity. Rewards and sanctions are fundamental manoeuvres that compel children into compliant 'good behaviour'. They require an engaged prefrontal cortex which can apply executive functioning and the capacity to stop and think. Reminding adults that difficult behaviours often arise out of a child's attempt at self-regulation, may result in them rethinking the use of sanctions that make no sense and cause a further rupture in their relationship with the child. You can't talk or persuade someone to feel safer.

Review Meetings and Endings

Review Meetings are necessary for the therapist to be able to evaluate therapeutic efficacy, re-examine therapeutic goals, review the number of therapy sessions offered, and provide ongoing psychoeducation. The CSECQ is designed to be used as an evaluation tool throughout the therapeutic process, as an additional lens through which therapeutic efficacy can be considered. From a polyvagal perspective, the therapist is interested in assessing whether the client can return to a ventral vagal position and is able to adaptively respond to their environment. As part of your review processes, you will be considering the following three questions: Can the child engage in developmentally appropriate social conversations? Are they able to play in a dynamic way, blending their social engagement system with either sympathetic or dorsal activation? Can they show appropriate intimacy with you, the toys, and/or others?

During the application of the CSECQ, the therapist and adult can revisit the polyvagal framework goals and explore whether the child has the capacity to:

- return to Ventral Vagal AWAKE State
- have an awareness of which State they are in
- adaptively move between autonomic states
- present an established Vagal Brake

As a shift in the child's regulatory capacity develops, the adult may present you with novel concerns or additional goals.

> As Emma's therapy progressed, she started to emerge from her existence in the AVOID State. In the therapy room Emma began using puppets to play out the experience of protesting or putting in boundaries, these behaviours started to become generalised at school and home. During a parental review meeting, Dawn noted that although Emma was still very quiet, she was coming out of her room more and spending time in communal spaces. She shared her surprise that Emma had "fronted up to her older sister and told her not to touch her stuff", sat down with everyone and changed the channel on the TV. Whilst Dawn was proud that Emma was able to put in this boundary for herself, she was concerned that Emma's behaviour would escalate, and she too would become "another angry child".
>
> Dawn was supported to reflect on whether Emma was autonomically reactive in response to her sister or had remained in a socially engaged position whilst putting in an appropriate boundary. Reminding Dawn to read Emma's physiological markers, tone of voice and facial expressions, she determined that whilst Emma might have been forceful, she had not become dysregulated.
>
> Indications from the review meeting suggested that Emma was beginning to be able to move between autonomic states and was starting to strengthen

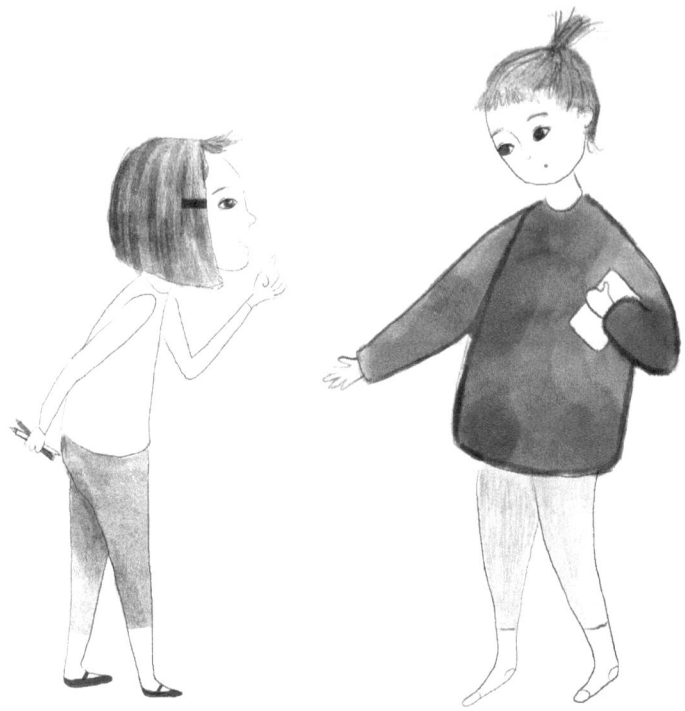

Figure 8.17 Emma defends herself.

her vagal tone. Ongoing therapy sessions would focus on broadening these positions for Emma, whilst also supporting her to develop her interoceptive awareness.

Endings

Concluding therapeutic sessions often elicits a range of emotional responses from everyone involved. Clients must say goodbye to a significant and trusted adult. Parents may experience heightened anxiety as they confront the perceived loss of a secure sanctuary for themselves. Teachers may feel they are once again left with the overall responsibility for the wellbeing of their students. The therapist must navigate the challenge of concluding their collaborative journey with a family, aware that they may never witness the unfolding chapters in that child's future. Involving parents and teachers in this significant decision early in the process offers the opportunity to gently end your relationship with them, whilst empowering them to be active participants in decisions about the child's wellbeing and future. Additionally, this involvement may foster a sense of agency and confidence in the adult, knowing that they have contributed to the decision-making process and are equipped to support the child's continued growth and development.

The way therapy concludes has a lasting impact on a child's perception of endings in relationships. Positive endings in therapy provide children with a template for secure relational closures, influencing how they approach and navigate endings in future interpersonal relationships. A therapist's ending with a child client, when approached with sensitivity and attunement, can have a ripple effect on the parents. Positive endings provide a model for secure relational closures and may contribute to a sense of safety within the family influencing parent-child dynamics. All align with the principles of the Polyvagal Theory in promoting co-regulation and social engagement.

The therapist was mindful that Ezra had a significant trauma history which was chronic and acute. Closure of therapeutic work had been discussed with Ezra and his parents, Elizabeth, and Jacob. The goal was to provide Ezra with an opportunity to end in a manner that would offer a new experience of loss. The ending was planned and paced as it was an integral part of his process. Symbolic Repair© afforded Ezra a reparative relationship of non-traumatic loss. Through the Polyvagal lens Ezra's sense of his world had become safe. The therapist had served as an attuned nervous system regulator which had supported the strengthening of Ezra's nervous system and ability to self-regulate. He was able to return quicker to the AWAKE State and no longer remained stuck in the ALARM State or AVOID State. At school Ezra was engaging more within his social engagement system, his body was responding through cues of safety cues rather than cues of danger. Energy was appropriate as it matched the situation and his body responded to danger when needed.

If the therapist ensures a smooth and positive ending for the child, it can contribute to the child's overall regulatory capacity. When parents perceive their child as being well-regulated and supported by the therapist, they may feel more confident in their own ability to regulate their child's emotions. This increased parental confidence can, in turn, positively influence the child's ongoing emotional development.

Chapter 9

Pandemic Hangover

Towards the end of 2019, a major health crisis was about to envelop the planet. It touched on every aspect of life and humanity. A social phenomenon like no other that quickly became known as the coronavirus disease 2019, more commonly as COVID-19.

Spreading across the world, the coronavirus became a global pandemic with most communities affected. Public health strategies were implemented in many countries, with the majority opting for extended periods of 'lockdown'. People who were identified as clinically extremely vulnerable or, were at a high risk of severe illness from COVID-19 were asked to shield by minimising contact with others. With unprecedented levels of need, there was a significant demand for health care, including child mental health services. Prolonged school closures had a major impact on learning for children. Key milestones and transitions were not marked or celebrated, with a lack of opportunity for them to connect with others, or to develop self-regulation skills.

Understanding the Coronavirus

A time of historical significance, SAR-CoV-19 emerged from China in late 2019, the World Health Organization (WHO) declaring it as a worldwide public health emergency, a 'pandemic of alarming levels of spread and severity' (2020). All countries to a lesser degree were impacted. The political landscape could often be seen as merging with the virus, exposing inequalities in health, socio-economic class, race, ethnicity, age, disability particularly apparent in the Western world.

Copious amounts of accurate and inaccurate information delivered on social media was termed as 'infodemic' by WHO (2020). Professionals and parents tried to navigate conflicting media coverage, which was creating, instilling, and reinforcing uncertainty, as it magnified all that was being experienced. Repetitive coverage of the pandemic crisis amplified visual and auditory sensory systems increasing psychological distress. Often like a tsunami, waves of emotional and mental reactions were experienced. The ability to manage everyday situations diminished. We have called this 'Social Media Trauma' and define it as: Social Media coverage that creates and controls a narrative of fear through an emotional and psychological lens which ultimately takes away an individual's decision making leading to paralysis of autonomy.

DOI: 10.4324/9781003412571-10

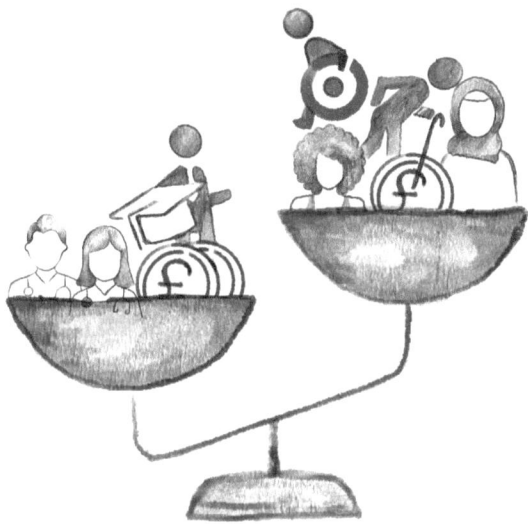

Figure 9.1 Inequalities.

To give context and for clarity, epidemic and pandemic are both Greek words. Both have several meanings but are often used in the context of disease. Epidemic can be applied to any situation that leads to a detrimental increase of health risks, whereas pandemic can be used to describe the rapid spread of a transmissible infection or communicable disease.

According to the Centers for Disease Control and Prevention (2012), epidemic refers to 'an increase, often sudden in the number of cases of a disease above what is normally expected in that area'. In comparison, pandemic refers to "an epidemic that has spread over several countries or continents, usually affecting a large number of people". In the context of COVID-19, WHO assessed that it could be characterised as a pandemic rather than an epidemic on 11 March 2020. Notably, the timeframe of most pandemics is 2–3 years, as viruses typically mutate and evolve with incidence and death rates reduced significantly.

Historically, Coronavirus was first described in 1967 from research carried out into the common cold. Published in the Journal of General Virology, the study involved nasal washings from over twenty volunteers. Cells were cultured for known viruses, and unexpectedly, an anomaly emerged, which had not previously been found in the human respiratory tract, identified as B814. Now known as HCoV-229E, viral imagining and subsequent findings showed that B814 belonged to a previously unrecognised group of viruses, which had certain characteristics. These include a petal shape rather than a sharp or pointed shape which were given the name coronaviruses. The spherical structure of coronaviruses is coated with spikes of protein, which the virus binds to causing healthy cells to be infected. It is worth noting that COVID-19 vaccines

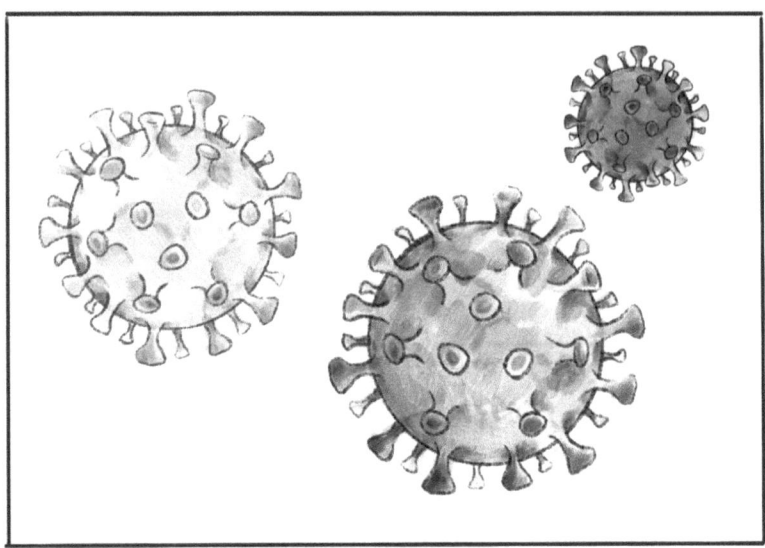

Figure 9.2 Coronavirus.

encourage the body to copy the spike protein to teach the immune system to attack it and fight the virus.

Highly contagious, SARS-CoV-2 is the virus that caused COVID-19 and is one of seven human coronaviruses that lead to respiratory difficulties including common cold infections in healthy adults. For those who have weak immune systems, there is the potential for long-term, life-threatening illnesses (Figure 9.3).

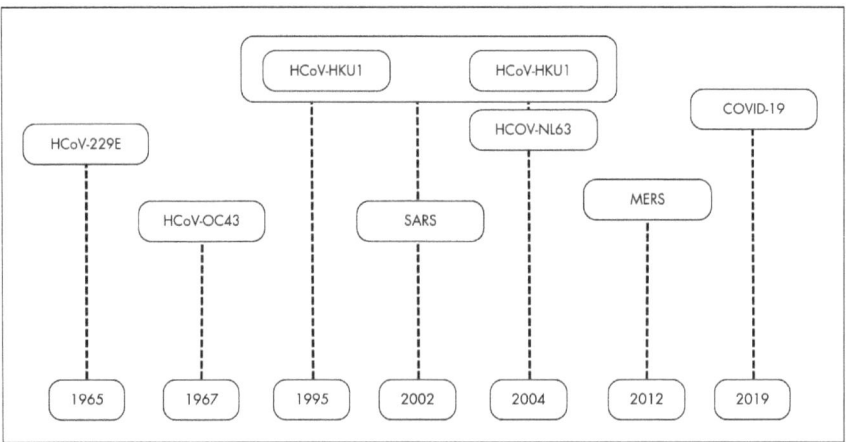

Figure 9.3 Coronavirus timeline.

It is believed that transmission of all seven human coronaviruses (HCoVs) has been from animals to humans. Three family members of the coronaviruses cause more severe illness; shortness of breath and severe acute respiratory disease, which sometimes results in death (Figure 9.4).

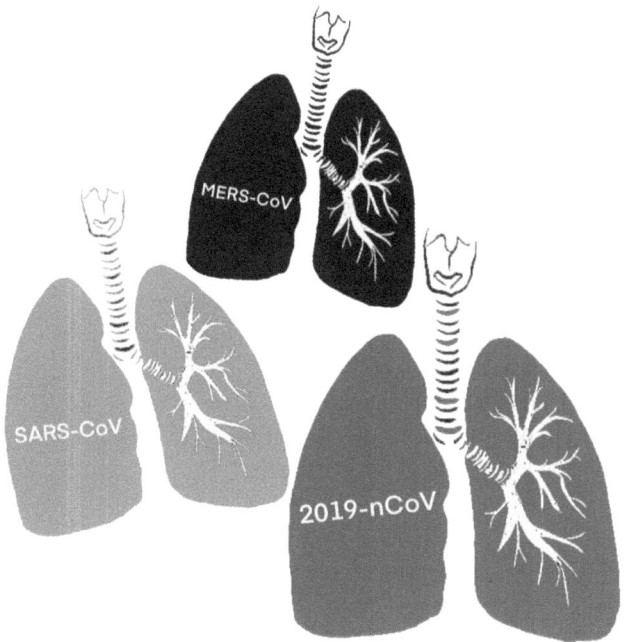

Figure 9.4 Lungs.

At the time of writing this book, there have been over 760 million global cases of COVID-19 and 6.9 million deaths (WHO, 2023), the actual number is thought to be higher.

Emerging evidence suggests that COVID-19 is a complex virus impacting on the body's immune system and inflammatory responses. Generally considered a respiratory illness, it involves the nervous system, including impaired concentration, depression, headaches, fatigue, vertigo, smell, taste. Moreover, the phenomenon of long COVID has emerged with over 65 million people experiencing symptoms two years post-COVID-19:

- Shortness of breath
- Heart-related difficulties; palpitations, chest pain, tightness
- Joint and muscle issues; pain, aches, pins, and needles
- Cognitive challenges; brain fog, memory, and concentration difficulties
- Sleeping difficulties; insomnia, daytime sleepiness
- Mental health issues; depression, anxiety, stress, fear

There is consensus amongst scientists that the coronavirus is here to stay. Globally, countries will need to adapt by making deliberate choices for societies to be able to live with the evolving nature and variations of this petal-shaped virus identified nearly seventy years ago.

Polyvagal Perspective: A Paradoxical Challenge

Known as the 'vagal paradox', Stephen Porges suggests that the vagus nerve is both a marker of resilience and a marker of risk factors. From a Polyvagal perspective, the coronavirus impacted on the autonomic nervous system of most human beings. Under siege from danger and crisis, physiologically, the human body was in a state of threat.

From an evolutionary perspective, human beings along with 4500 species are classified as mammals who share in four distinctive features:

- Fur/hair growing from the skin
- Mammary glands for producing milk
- Three bones in the middle ear to transmit sound to the inner ear
- Single bone on both sides of the lower jaw

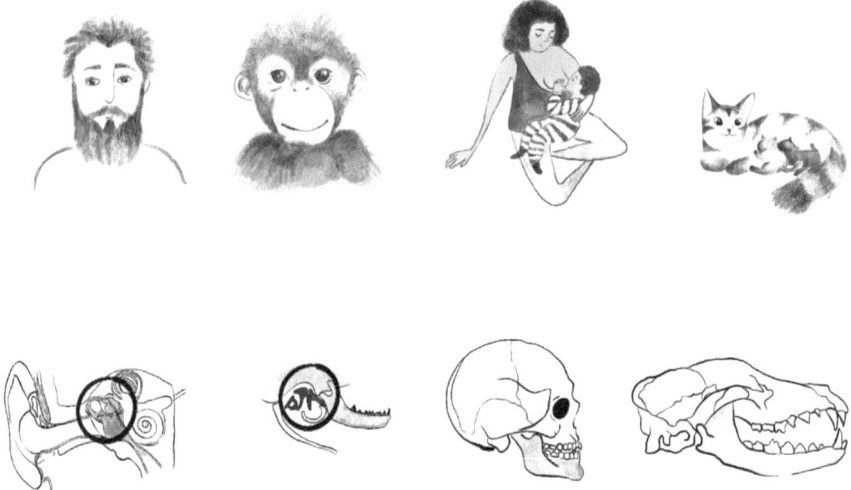

Figure 9.5 Mammalian features.

As primates, walking fully upright, the human brain has the largest number of cortical neurons with a cerebral cortex that supports complex, higher thinking, executive control, decision making, emotional regulation, language. Although the human body has evolved to respond to tolerate stress, it is not designed to handle chronic stress especially one that lasts three years and beyond.

During the pandemic, the average stress that people usually tolerate was pushed to the limit. People were living in a stress bucket 24/7, which amplified issues and impacted on the way in which the brain was able to solve problems.

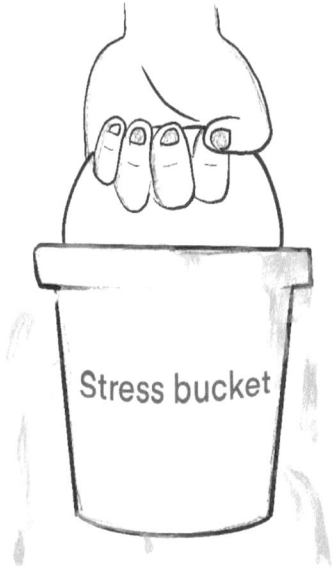

Figure 9.6 Stress bucket.

As the coronavirus is a fear stimulus, amygdala activation prepared the body to react to the danger of COVID-19 by increasing the hypothalamic-pituitary-adrenal axis (HPA). Known as the stress pathway, the hypothalamus causes the HPA to trigger the release of cortisol. As stress starts to build, the adrenal glands come under immense pressure. The body reacts with a fight or flight response, which directs the shutdown of non-vital bodily functions increasing vital bodily functions, including heart rate, blood pressure, and breathing rate. This can lead to the adrenal glands becoming weaker until they can tolerate no more stress. Given this context and that the ANS is biased in service of survival, it was impossible to 'convince' the nervous system that it was safe to move towards play, health, growth, and restoration.

The paradox of chronic stress is that it puts a person in a problem-solving mode, but our brain is unable to focus or take action. We are essentially put into a freeze position, with no capacity for productivity.

Through a trauma lens, it could be argued that COVID-19 was a collective trauma causing psychological injuries. Reflective of a disaster response, the pandemic could be associated with the emotional phases of trauma with survival systems in constant activation trying to protect us. Humans emotionally reacted in the context of an unsafe environment with the ANS stuck in a cycle of behaviours, thoughts, and feelings reacting to here and now events.

Familiar structures of boundaries, predictability, expectations disappeared with a fear of the unknown and sense of safety compromised. A surge in hormones heightened alertness and redistribution of blood to muscles prepared us for survival.

Ever present, the pandemic cloud provided the 'perfect' climate of toxic stress to the danger that was being experienced every day (Figure 9.7).

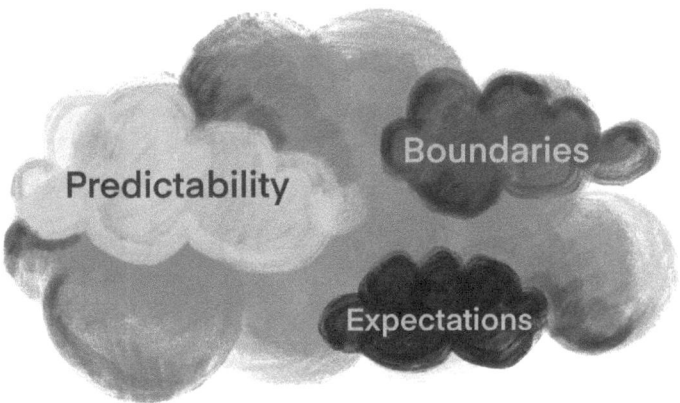

Figure 9.7 Pandemic cloud.

Through a polyvagal lens, we see that modulation between the parasympathetic system and sympathetic nervous system needed to bring the ANS to homeostasis was limited. This was due to rapid shifting and moving of hierarchy, ventral vagal into sympathetic and dorsal states. Forced isolation meant that there was lack of opportunity to discharge the energy from within the sympathetic nervous system causing it to be lodged within the body, stuck in a trauma response.

During this period, Deb Dana (2023) suggests that three autonomic needs for safety were constantly being tested: context, choice, connection.

Context: The autonomic nervous system is a state response. It needs information and context to make sense of what is happening and to feel reassured. If this does not happen, the brain will create a story to reflect the individual's perceptions based on information inside (body), outside (environment), and in-between (people) to support nervous and autonomic connection and safety.

Choice: If the nervous system feels that it has little choice or feels trapped, it enacts a nervous system survival response. During COVID-19, choices were limited, bringing about either a sympathetic fight or flight (mobilised) response or dorsal/disconnect (shutdown/despair) response.

Connection: Essential for the nervous system to feel safe enough to engage in the world from a regulated place, throughout the pandemic, connection was reduced, restricted, or taken away. New ways had to be found to attend to the nervous system and support safety and regulation. In many households, where possible, engagement happened through online platforms.

Continual threat of the virus and social distancing measures prevented the move towards a place of calm. For children, the ability of their caregiver to effectively co-regulate and support states of arousal or modify emotions, thoughts, and behaviours was thwarted due to lack of opportunity for safe proximal relationships. Simultaneously, there was also a silent mental health pandemic. Prolonged lockdowns and social distancing served as barriers to relational experiences. Safe Harbours were lost. Basic anchors were not in place and finding a way back home to Ventral was almost impossible due to looping and being trapped in Sympathetic or Dorsal distress.

Amira was a much-wanted baby for Layla and Ali. Amira's mum was 4 months pregnant at the start of the pandemic. Pregnancy related checks were on-line, and Layla saw very few professionals. Throughout pregnancy Layla was fearful

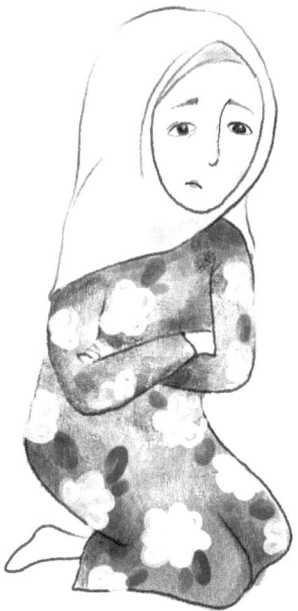

Figure 9.8 Layla.

that something would happen to her unborn baby. Layla did not want to con-nect with people and the outside world. For the rest of her pregnancy and until the present day, she came to believe that family members, other people, and environments where she had previously felt safe, were dangerous and continue to be. We see that Layla's autonomic needs for context, choice and safety have been compromised. Her body's response has been of Dorsal disconnect and she appears to be in AVOID State, stuck in a trauma response.

School Disruption

As every individual is unique with their own reality of the pandemic, it could be argued that there is no universal experience of the pandemic. Nevertheless, we know that the instability of COVID-19 was a psychological burden especially to children. Well-being was negatively affected with worsening mental health and behaviours due to quarantine measures. Enforced lockdowns impacted on opportunities to socialise, play, and learn.

Although children were at a low health physical risk from COVID-19, emerging data about the psychological impact on them was, and continues to be, concerning. Disruption to their lives presented immeasurable challenges that exposed them to significant risk factors for mental health issues. Whilst some thrived, many did not. Of those who didn't, their well-being and mental health was significantly affected. School closures, social isolation, economic instability, and health anxiety led to psychological distress and behaviours, which continue for many.

Teddy was isolated in lockdown as his grandparents were shielding due to their health needs. Teddy has struggled to go back to nursery. His grandma states that "there are more problems with Teddy and his behaviour than before the lock-downs". Betty grapples to get him into nursery. There are days where his 'melt-downs' are so big she feels that she has no choice but to take him home rather than battling with his behavioural distress in the nursery playground. We see that Teddy's ANS is responding to cues of danger when in the nursery setting. He moves into a mobilised state of sympathetic activation. Through a trauma lens, when Teddy's grandma attempts to drop him off at nursery, he is triggered by feelings of abandonment which he likely experienced on numerous occasions with Jemma, his mum. He cannot distinguish between past experiences and feel-ings in the present of being 'abandoned'. He becomes aroused and is in the ALARM State. Teddy needs co-regulation which his grandma provides for him. In her presence, Teddy eventually returns to the AWAKE State.

Impact on Services

Services and professionals working across a range of disciplines with children were stretched beyond the limit. All presented significant challenges for governments, voluntary, and private sector organisations. Sudden implementations of restrictions meant that in-person communications were limited, and traditional face-to-face interactions moved to virtual overnight.

There were differences in how countries responded to COVID-19. The UK government introduced a series of temporary changes to Children's Social Care regulations, relaxing a range of duties relating to children in care. On 25 March 2020, the Coronavirus Act introduced a range of measures to the Care Act, 2014 in England, and the Social Services and Well-being (Wales) Act 2014. This was done 'to enable local authorities to prioritise the services they offer in order to ensure the most urgent and serious care needs are met, even if this means not meeting everyone's assessed needs in full or delaying some assessments' (Department of Health and Social Care, 2020). Local Authorities, safeguarding and regulated partners were asked to work within the statutory framework. However, due to social distancing measures, many services were suspended or reduced with face-to-face support limited. In addition, support mechanisms in the National Health Service (NHS), including child and adolescent mental health services, and hospital outpatient clinics, were closed, suspended, or moved to virtual home-based clinics.

Ezra had been booked to have a planned procedure for tightening of scars to his feet from his burn injury. His mobility had been severely impacted and the hope was that the surgery would help with his movement. Ezra's surgery was postponed, his parents had been advised that due to waiting lists there will be at least 12 months delay. In addition, Ezra's play therapy stopped during the pandemic and his therapist, whom he worked with long-term, had retired. Ezra is using his wheelchair more at school, becoming increasingly angry. When this happens, the school risk assessment states that the classroom must be evacuated, as it is deemed that he is at risk to others. He is left alone to 'calm down'. Ezra uses his upper body to express himself, throwing his walking sticks and anything else that is in his way. We see that Ezra moves towards high sympathetic arousal into ALARM State. A trauma response might be activated when Ezra is left alone with his big feelings. This may trigger his body memory of being left when he sustained his burn injury (if only for a few minutes), as he screamed and flailed in his distress as a one-year-old.

According to Save the Children, the pandemic caused extraordinary disruption to children's education and at its height, 1.6 billion children and young people were out of school: approximately 90% of the entire student population (June 2020). School closures and remote learning became the norm with "governments mandating that schools be closed, and that education be delivered remotely" (UNESCO, 2021).

Schools and early years provisions in the UK were closed from 23 March 2020 to all pupils except vulnerable children or those whose caregivers were critical workers. All other children were required to access remote learning from home. Even though schools partially opened on 1 June 2020, most school-aged children did not return to education until the beginning of the new academic year in September 2020.

Moreover, data from Ofcom (2020) highlights digital exclusion pre-pandemic of school-aged children in the UK. The data shows that children already disadvantaged due to social and demographic factors (socio-demographics) resulted in digital inequality of education throughout the pandemic. Inequalities in access to learning were also dependent on the availability and support of the parent, teacher, and school. Data also shows that children in lower earning households were more affected by these issues.

With restrictions gradually lifted, there was a transition back to face-to-face learning. However, there is a consensus that the pandemic seems to have been a main driver in the decline of pupil behaviour. As school returners have re-engaged in education, teachers have noticed an increase in mental health challenges and behaviours. With permanent closures, suspensions, or reduced child and mental health services, schools are struggling with the negative impact of the pandemic on pupil well-being and behaviour:

- Immaturity
- Lack of confidence; more cautious, less willing to take risks
- Poor social skills; lack of engagement
- Violence; aggressions towards staff
- Academic underachievement; apathy
- School dropout

Arrested Development and Risk

Emerging data from studies pre and post pandemic suggest that mental health was worse for some children but improved for others. Dependent on age, gender, ethnicity, class, disability, support networks, and socio-economic factors, distress experienced has been multifaceted. Observed symptoms include:

- Depression, fatigue
- Stress, anxiety, worry
- Fear, anger
- Boredom, loneliness
- Disrupted sleep

For many children, there were considerable risks at home and online with many vulnerable to child criminal exploitation, child sexual exploitation, radicalisation, and violence. Alongside Adverse Childhood Experiences, there were also:

- Disruptions to areas of child development
- Post-traumatic stress disorder
- Sexual violence
- Crime
- Trafficking
- Child marriage

Other horrific consequences for children and young people have included:

- Family disintegration
- Family economic hardship
- Institutionalisation

There is a growing body of evidence from studies that a lack of exposure and interacting with people has significantly impacted babies and children. Research studies from Rhode Island Hospital and the non-profit LENA Foundation (2020) highlight the impact on babies born during the pandemic. Their data shows that vocalisation and engagement in verbal interactions was less in comparison to those born pre-pandemic.

In a small-scale study published by the British Medical Journal (2022), findings showed that babies screened at six months using the Ages and Stages Questionnaire (developmental screening tool) in comparison to those born pre-pandemic scored slightly lower in areas related to motor and social skills but not in areas related to communication or problem-solving skills. The same study suggested that COVID-19 related maternal stress experienced during pregnancy may be one reason that explains the difference in developmental delays.

A study of 887 children in Japan: 447 children aged 1–3 years and 440 children aged 3–5 years, who were exposed to the pandemic found that they were 4.39 months behind in development age at 5 years (JAMA Pediatrics, July, 2023).

Amira is 12 months old. There are concerns about Layla's connection with Amira. Professionals involved with the family have identified that Amira is not meeting her developmental milestones and that her needs are not being met by her parents. She has been described as a 'smiley baby' who rarely cries. Amira has never been taken to parent-baby groups and has not had the opportunity for social interaction and stimulation. In front of professionals, Amira presents as a baby who seeks co-regulation. Her vagal tone may be underdeveloped because she has had minimal contact with anybody outside her family home or experiences to practice utilising her ventral brake.

A UK research study by The Institute of Fiscal Studies (2023) surveyed 6095 parents living in England with children aged 4–16 years: 'How did parents' experiences in the labour market shape children's social and emotional development during the pandemic?'

- 47% of parents reported that their child had more socio-emotional difficulties in 2021 than the year before
- 52% of children aged 4–7 years in comparison to those aged 12–15 years were 10% more likely to have worsened social and emotional development
- Furloughed parents of girls reported worsening socio-emotional skill in their child in comparison to children of parents who had stable employment

Adult deaths from COVID-19 have meant that many children are bereft or orphaned with huge consequences for their short-term and long-term future. A study published in JAMA Paediatrics (May, 2022) estimates that 10.5 million children under the age of eighteen years have experienced the death of a parent or caregiver. Of these, 7.5 million are orphaned with the highest number of deaths in South-east Asia and African Regions.

Emerging evidence suggests that the pandemic will lead to the same potential outcomes as traditional ACEs. For many children, there will be an impact on their health and well-being across the life continuum.

Teletherapy

Teletherapy, also known as telepsychology, is "psychological counselling or psychotherapy by videoconferencing, text messaging, e-mail or telephone" (https://dicitonary.com).

In response to COVID-19 and the global pandemic, most therapists needed to quickly adapt and find ways to continue to offer therapy in an ever-changing landscape. Many concerns, questions, and worries were expressed, combined with huge anxiety as to how to maintain connection with clients through a two-dimensional platform whilst being authentic and having presence through the screen. Therapeutically, with so many disruptions to routines and structure, there was a need for therapists to bridge their own ANS 'A' States and lean into their social engagement system to transfer safety and connection to online working. For many children, teletherapy was a lifeline during chaos and fear.

Therapists were aware of the importance of maintaining continuity for the client especially as they had lost so many other connections. Demand was significant due to increased needs in mental health with therapists and clients entering a new era of how therapy was offered and accessed, respectively. Some therapists felt distanced by the screen, whilst others felt able to reach their clients with a feeling of connectedness. Predominantly, therapists had to jump into the realms of the unknown as using teletherapy was an unfamiliar way of working. For those who had experience of using video conferencing platforms, they embraced the technologies with confidence and a knowing.

In the first few months, it was 'as if' there was a developmental regression for some therapists as they tried something new, having to quickly learn and grow from the experience. Guidance, support, and advice were sought with governments and professional bodies regulating where and how teletherapy could be offered.

Environmental challenges presented themselves within the context of an unfamiliar therapeutic space as both therapist and client were invited into each other's homes. Video platforms, Wi-Fi connections, intrusion of noises, children and animals wandering in and out, views of ceilings, floors, walls, furniture. The list is endless!

In the context of the Polyvagal Theory, therapists had to hold and contain their own anxiety and personal experiences of COVID-19, aware of the importance of stepping into their own State of regulation and safety to be a regulating resource for clients. For those clients who were transferring from face-to-face to online, it was often easier as the therapeutic relationship had been established and there was a familiarity with each other's nervous systems. More challenging was working with new clients, as there had not been the luxury of the intimacy of face-to-face experiences.

A developmental piece, teletherapy was a growth process with bumps along the way. Learning the art of intimacy and broadcasting cues of safety rather than cues of danger was often about the therapist's ability to trust in the process. There was a need to take time to find the pace of the conversation with the client, which was very different through a screen. Bringing features of face-to-face therapy to the online experience brought its own challenge. Using the two-dimensional modality of a screen, whilst regulating the client, was often more tiring. There was a need to pay attention to the environment and maintain an 'intimate' experience for the client through voice prosody, gestures, moving back and forth into the camera, as a way of compensating for a lack of face-to-face interactions.

Flexibility, going with the flow, and modelling the courage to be imperfect was all part of expanding the window of tolerance for therapist and client. Projecting authentic presence was vital for the client to feel contained. There was a need for therapists to be anchored in the AWAKE State, lending themselves across and through the camera to help clients move within their hierarchal States of arousal. Many of us felt like novices. Confidence meant leaning into the therapeutic relationship in a different way and trusting in the connection. We tried to maintain connectedness by engaging our social engagement system to support intimacy of the therapeutic work online.

Emerging from the intensity of COVID-19, many therapists have chosen to exclusively offer teletherapy rather than return to face-to-face work. There has been a need for therapists to contain and manage client feelings through the screen and incorporate a range of techniques to support social engagement to regulate the ANS and achieve therapeutic goals. From a Polyvagal and therapeutic perspective, this can be perceived as the autonomic nervous system projecting on the conscious mind as it seeks healthy homeostasis.

Key to supporting hyper-aroused and hypo-aroused states are experiences of co-regulation to support homeostatic functioning to modify emotions, thoughts, behaviours. Lockdowns and social distancing served as barriers to co-regulation. In addition, often the ability for the caregiver to effectively co-regulate their child was difficult because of their own feelings of overwhelm and stress. Thus, the instinctual drive to calm through safe proximal relationships was hindered.

Biologically, the phenomenon of COVID-19 was a pressing time for nervous systems as there was a generalised neuroception of threat. In a world that was imploding, the ANS was trying to serve in the best way it could, by moving towards the foundational level of survival and maintaining a state of body hypervigilance.

Whilst there remains continued uncertainty about the long-term effects for children, especially those born at the height of the pandemic who are known as 'pandemic babies' (early 2020 onwards), there are glimmers. As we move towards a post COVID-19 era, we see that there are some positive changes and that faced with adversity, resilience has been highlighted in some aspects of our lives.

Chapter 10

Healing through a Polyvagal Lens

A Polyvagal Informed Approach to Therapeutic Work with Children and Young People offers therapists a broader perspective from which to approach their work with children. Extending our frame of reference through a Polyvagal lens gives additional insight into the neurobiological roots of discordant behaviours and attachment strategies. This knowledge empowers therapists to tailor interventions that promote safety, co-regulation, and ultimately, the development of healthier nervous system functioning in children. By integrating the Polyvagal Theory into their practice, therapists can enhance their ability to foster secure attachments, mitigate trauma responses, and facilitate emotion regulation, ultimately leading to more effective therapeutic outcomes.

Delving deeper into the practical applications of a polyvagal framework supports practitioners to consider how neurobiological mechanisms outlined in the theory can inform specific therapeutic techniques and interventions. In paying attention to physiological markers signalling signs of dysregulation in the nervous system of our clients, strategies can be implemented to help them regulate their emotions and behaviours more effectively. Through exploring how to better foster a safe and supportive therapeutic environment, a felt sense of safety and connection will be promoted, facilitating healing and growth. By expanding our understanding of the Polyvagal Theory, we can enhance our ability to provide targeted and effective interventions that address the unique needs of our young clients.

Many therapists working with children and young people utilise play, metaphor and creativity as a vehicle for change. The Polyvagal Theory cements our understanding of the importance of play. We learn that it is a neural exercise, directly influencing the development and regulation of the autonomic nervous system. Playful interactions provide a safe and engaging environment, activating the AWAKE State. Through play, children learn to modulate their physiological responses, navigating between the ANS 'A' States (AWAKE, ALARM, and AVOID). This process promotes the strengthening and flexibility of neural pathways associated with social connection and emotion regulation, contributing to the development of the vagal brake, adaptive stress responses and secure attachment bonds. Through maintaining an optimised window of tolerance and utilising Symbolic Repair©,

DOI: 10.4324/9781003412571-11

clients can experience the adaptive blending of the ANS 'A' States. By recognising play as a neural exercise, therapists can harness its transformative power to support children's emotional well-being and neurodevelopmental growth.

Applying a Polyvagal framework insists on therapists having an awareness of their own autonomic responses and attending to their needs as they arise. Work with children principally involves right brain to right brain, non-verbal communication. This invites us to take on the somatic experiences of our clients. We must remain alert to the potential dysregulation in our own nervous systems. A dysregulated adult cannot offer co-regulation.

Familiarising ourselves with the potential triggers, which move us into taking defensive action in the ALARM State or hide us in the AVOID State, provides a profound sense of empowerment. It is also key to shielding ourselves from burnout. Therapeutic work is intense, and we need to know the circumstances, actions, sounds, thoughts, or emotions that lead to involuntarily defensive reactions. We also need to know what serves our return to homeostasis, not only for our own benefit but also to demonstrate regulation-in-action, sparking our client's mirror neurons and showing them the way.

This is especially relevant for our work with children who present with adaptive responses formed in threatening environments. Their perception of threat persists even when the threat has been removed, presenting a paradoxical challenge in therapeutic intervention. The case of a withdrawn child, whose autonomic response remains defensive despite the presence of a caring therapist, exemplifies this enduring conflict between past survival mechanisms and present opportunities for connection.

Moving forward, The Needs Paradox® framework offers a valuable perspective on navigating the psychobiological complexities inherent in therapeutic care for trauma-affected children. Recognising the protective adaptations developed by these children, therapists play a crucial role in delicately balancing the repair of original wounds with the validation and respect of survival strategies. Through interventions informed by Polyvagal Theory, therapists can repeatedly signal safety to recalibrate the autonomic nervous system and foster a sense of security necessary for healing.

The Physiological Marker Checklist© (PMC) and Child Social Engagement Capacity Questionnaire© (CSECQ) are designed to enhance therapists' case conceptualisation. Utilising both these tools will ensure that a polyvagal lens is incorporated into the formulation process. Using the CSECQ in your meetings with parents and teachers can be a good starting point for offering Polyvagal Theory concepts. These can be developed further with the use of The Super Protector© and additional activities offered throughout the book.

A Polyvagal Informed Approach to Therapeutic Work with Children and Young People is intended to bolster therapeutic work regardless of the modality or approach taken. By applying concepts from the Polyvagal Theory, therapists have a more expansive vista and can make sense of behaviours and responses that were once perplexing. Sharing this information with clients, their teachers and parents takes away judgement and shame, providing a pathway to healing.

At its core, a Polyvagal approach to therapy is rooted in the understanding that safety and trusted connections are fundamental to human existence. Through this lens, we hold absolute respect for the necessary adaptations our clients have made in response to past experiences, reflecting their innate drive for self-preservation. By embracing this theory, therapists can embark on a journey to support their clients in cultivating trust, resilience, and a playful curiosity for life. This ultimately fosters an integrated self, capable of thriving in relationships and navigating life's challenges.

Bibliography

Almeida, J. D., & Tyrrell, D. A. (1967). The Morphology of Three Previously Uncharacterized Human Respiratory Viruses That Grow in Organ Culture. *Journal of General Virology*, April;1(2), 175–178. https://doi.org/10.1099/0022-1317-1-2-175

American Academy of Pediatrics (2014). *Adverse Childhood Experiences and the Lifelong Consequences of Trauma*. Elk Grove Village, IL: AAP.

Ammann, R. (1991). *Healing and Transformation in Sandplay*. La Salle: Open Court Publishing Company.

Auger, F. V. (2016). *Neurobiological dimensions of transference/countertransference interpreted through the lend of analytical psychology and modern physics*. Saybrook University ProQuest Dissertations Publishing.

Badenoch, B. (2018a). "Safety Is the Treatment". In S. W. Porges & D. Dana (Eds.), *Clinical Applications of the Polyvagal Theory: The Emergence of Polyvagal-Informed Therapies* (pp. 73–88). New York: W. W. Norton & Company.

Badenoch, B. (2018b). *The Heart of Trauma: Healing the Embodied Brain in the Context of Relationships*. London: W. W. Norton & Company.

Barnes, M. (2013). *The Healing Path with Children*. Uckfield: Play Therapy Press Limited.

Beauchaine, T. P., Gatzke-Kopp, L., & Mead, H. K. (2007). Polyvagal Theory and Developmental Psychopathology: Emotion Dysregulation and Conduct Problems from Preschool to Adolescence. *Biological Psychology*, 74(2), 174–184. https://doi.org/10.1016/j.biopsycho.2005.08.008

Bellis, M. A., Hughes, K., & Leckenby, N. et al. (2014). National Household Survey of Adverse Childhood Experiences and Their Relationship with Resilience to Health-Harming Behaviors in England. *BMC Medicine*, 12, 72. https://doi.org/10.1186/1741-7015-12-72

Böhmer, M. (2010). "Communication by Impact" and Other Forms of Non-Verbal Communication: A Review of Transference, Countertransference and Projective Identification. *African Journal of Psychiatry*, 13, 179–183.

Bowers, M. E., & Yehuda, R. (2016). Intergenerational Transmission of Stress in Humans. *Neuropsychopharmacology: Official Publication of the American College of Neuropsychopharmacology*, 41(1), 232–244. https://doi.org/10.1038/npp.2015.247

Bowlby, J. (1951). Maternal Care and Mental Health. *Bulletin of the World Health Organization*, 3, 355–533.

Bowlby, J. (1988). *A Secure Base: Parent-Child Attachment and Healthy Human Development*. New York: Basic Books.

British Medical Journal (2022). Covid-19: Babies Born During the Pandemic Show Slight Development Delays. *BMJ*, 2022, 376. https://doi.org/10.1136/bmj.o29

Bromberg, P. M. (2006). *Awakening the Dreamer: Clinical Journey*. Mahwah, NJ: Analytic Press.

Busuttil, W. (2009). Complex Post-traumatic Stress Disorder: A Useful Diagnostic Framework? *Psychiatry.* https://doi.org/10.1016/j.mppsy.2009.04.014

Cadogan, S. (2016) *An Exploration of the Use of Sand as a Medium in Psychotherapy with Adults.* [Online]. MA in Psychotherapy. Dublin Business School, School of Arts (Unpublished)

Center on the Developing Child at Harvard University. (2015). *Resilience*, viewed 13 April 2023, https://developingchild.harvard.edu/science/key-concepts/resilience/

Centers for Disease Control and Prevention (CDC). (2012). Principles of Epidemiology in Public Health Practice, Third Edition. *Lesson 1: Introduction to Epidemiology* Waldorf: PHF Publication Sales. https://www.cdc.gov/csels/dsepd/ss1978/lesson1/section11.html

Cerritelli, F., Frasch, M. G., Antonelli, M. C., Viglione, C., Vechhi, S., Chiera, M., & Manzotti, A. (20 September 2021) Review on the Vagus Nerve and Autonomic Nervous System During Fetal Development: Searching for Critical Windows. *Frontiers in Neuroscience*, 15, | https://doi.org/10.3389/fnins.2021.721605

Cherland, E. (2012). The Polyvagal Theory: Neurophysiological Foundations of Emotions, Attachment, Communication, Self-Regulation. *Journal of the Canadian Academy of Child and Adolescent Psychiatry*, 21(4), 313–314.

Child Welfare Information Gateway. (2006). Understanding the Effects of Maltreatment on Early Brain Development. Available at: http://ngolearning.com.au/files/face2face-courses/CP-dynamics/Understandingtheeffectsofmaltreatmentonbraindevelopment.pdf

Childhood Adversity Team (2021) *Adverse Childhood Experiences (ACEs)* viewed on 13 April 2023, https://www.healthscotland.scot/population-groups/children/adverse-childhood-experiences-aces/should-services-ask-about-aces

Cook, R., Bird, G., Catmur, C., Press, C., & Heyes, C. (2014). Mirror Neurons: From Origin to Function. *Behavioral and Brain Sciences*, 37(2), 177–192. https://doi.org/10.1017/S0140525X13000903

Coronavirus: COVID-19, Changes to the Care Act 2014 https://www.gov.uk/government/publications/coronavirus-COVID-19-changes-to-the-care-act-2014/care-act-easements-guidance-for-local-authorities

Cozolino, L. (2006). *The Neuroscience of Human Relationships*. London: W. W. Norton & Company.

Cozolino, L. J. (2004). *The Making of a Therapist: A Practical Guide for the Inner Journey*. New York: W. W. Norton.

Dahlen, A. I. (2022). Teaching through a Polyvagal Lens: Using the Science of Safety to Co-Regulate in the Classroom. Master's thesis, Bethel University. Spark Repository. https://spark.bethel.edu/etd/908

Damasio, A. (2003). *Looking for Spinoza: Joy, Sorrow, and the Feeling Brain*. Orlando, FL: Harcourt, Inc.

Damasio, A. R. (1994). *Descartes' Error: Emotion, Reason, and the Human Brain*. New York: G. P. Putman's Sons.

Dana, D. (2018). *The Polyvagal Theory in Therapy: Engaging the Rhythm of Regulation*. London: W. W. Norton & Company.

Dana, D. (2023). *Polyvagal-Informed Practitioner Online Course: Proven Interventions to Guide Clients Toward Safety and Connection.* https://www.pesi.co.uk/sales/uk_c_001951_polyvagalpractitioner_organic-813508?srsltid=AfmBOorAHZaYePhANT37BMG87oaAT3Ge3PlqfYSnKjZlFPa0Une9PCog

Daniel, S., & Trevarthen, C. (2017). *Rhythms of Relating in Children's Therapies: Connecting Creatively with Vulnerable Children*. London: Jessica Kingsley Publishers.

Department of Health and Social Care. (2020). https://www.gov.uk/organisations

Diamond, L. M., Fagundes, C. P., & Butterworth, M. R. (2011). *Attachment Style, Vagal Tone, and Empathy During Mother–Adolescent Interactions. Journal of Research on Adolescence*, 22(1), 165–184.

Digiuseppe, R., Linscott, J., & Jilton, R.. (1996). *Developing the Therapeutic Alliance in Child—adolescent Psychotherapy. Applied and Preventive Psychology*, 5, 85–100. 10.1016/S0962-1849(96)80002-3.

Dijk, W. 2023, Insecure attachment: What can the polyvagal theory add to your life? Accessed on 19 January 2023. Available at: https://madinthenetherlands-org.translate.goog/onveilige-hechting-polyvagaal-theorie/?_x_tr_sl=auto&_x_tr_tl=en&_x_tr_hl=en&_x_tr_pto=wapp

Dion, L. (2018). *Aggression in Play Therapy: A Neurobiological Approach for Integrating Intensity*. New York: W. W. Norton & Company.

Dion, L. (2021). *Neuroception of Safety: Not Always What We Think*. Available at: https://synergeticplaytherapy.com/neuroception-of-safety-not-always-what-we-think/

Dönmez, A., & Ceylan, M. (2013). The Neurobiology of Transference. *Journal of Mind & Behavior*, 34, 233–258.

Else, P. (2009). *The Value of Play*. London: Continuum.

Erikson, E. H. (1963). *Youth: Change and Challenge*. London: Basic books.

Faust, K. M., Carouso-Peck, S., Elson, M. R., & Goldstein, M. H. (2020). The Origins of Social Knowledge in Altricial Species. *Annual Review of Developmental Psychology*, 2, 225–246. https://doi.org/10.1146/annurev-devpsych-051820-121446

Field, T., & Diego, M. (2008). Vagal Activity, Early Growth and Emotional Development. *Infant Behavior & Development*, 31(3), 361–373. https://doi.org/10.1016/j.infbeh.2007.12.008

Fonagy, P., Steele, M., Steele, H., Moran, G. S., & Higgitt, A. C. (1991). The Capacity for Understanding Mental States: The Reflective Self in Parent and Child and Its Significance for Security of Attachment. *Infant Mental Health Journal*, 12(3), 201–218. https://doi.org/10.1002/1097-0355(199123)12:3<201::AID-IMHJ2280120307>3.0.CO;2-7

Fonagy, P., & Target, M. (2005). Bridging the Transmission Gap: An End to an Important Mystery of Attachment Research? *Attachment & Human Development*, 7(3), 333–343. https://doi.org/10.1080/14616730500269278

Ford, K., Barton, E., Newbury, A., Hughes, K., Bezeczky, Z., Roderick, J., & Bellis, M. (2019). *Understanding the Prevalence of Adverse Childhood Experiences (ACEs) in a Male Offender Population in Wales: The Prisoner ACE Survey*. Public Health Wales; Bangor University.

Fuchs, T. (2004). Neurobiology and Psychotherapy: an Emerging Dialogue. *Current Opinion in Psychology*, 17, 479–485. https://doi.org/10.1097/00001504-200411000-00010

Gallese, V. (2009). Mirror Neurons, Embodied Simulation, and the Neural Basis of Social Identification. *Psychoanalytic Dialogues*, 19(5), 519–536. https://doi.org/10.1080/10481880903231910

Gallese, V. (2014). Bodily Selves in Relation: Embodied Simulation as Second-Person Perspective on Intersubjectivity. *Philosophical Transactions of the Royal Society of London. Series B, Biological Sciences*, 369(1644), 20130177. https://doi.org/10.1098/rstb.2013.0177

Gardner, D., & Harper, P. (1997). "Using Metaphor and Imagery". In K. N. Dwivedi (Ed.), *The Therapeutic Use of Stories* (pp. 100–111). London: Routledge.

Gaskill, R. L., & Perry, B. D. (2014). "The Neurobiological Power of Play: Using the Neurosequential Model of Therapeutics to Guide Play in the Healing Process". In C. A. Malchiodi & D. A. Crenshaw (Eds.), *Creative Arts and Play Therapy for Attachment Problems* (pp. 178–194). New York: The Guilford Press

Geller, S. M., & Porges, S. W. (2014). Therapeutic Presence: Neurophysiological Mechanisms Mediating Feeling Safe in Therapeutic Relationships. *Journal of Psychotherapy Integration*, 24(3), 178–192. https://doi.org/10.1037/a0037511

Gendlin, E.T. 1978. *Focusing*. 1st ed. New York: Everest House

Giano, Z., Wheeler, D. L., & Hubach, R. D. (2020). The Frequencies and Disparities of Adverse Childhood Experiences in the U.S. *BMC Public Health*, 20, 1327. https://doi.org/10.1186/s12889-020-09411-z

Gil, E. (2006) Helping Abused and Traumatized Children: Integrating Directive and Non-directive Approaches. In C. A. Malchiodi (Ed.), *Creative Interventions with Traumatized Children* (pp. 178–194). New York: The Guilford Press.

Goodyear-Brown, P. (2019). *Trauma and Play Therapy: Helping Children Heal*. London: Routledge.

Gordon, T. J. (2018). Utilizing Animal Metaphors in Child Psychotherapy: An Integrative Approach for Therapists. *The Graduate Review*, 3, 135–148.

Gross, S. (2021). "Linguistic Judgments as Evidence". In N. Allott, T. Lohndal & G. Rey (Eds.), *A Companion to Chomsky* (pp. 544–556). Hoboken, NJ: Wiley Blackwell.

Hadiprodjo, N. (2018) *Clinical applications of the Polyvagal Theory and Attachment theory to Play Therapy for Children with Developmental Trauma*. Doctoral Thesis. University of Roehampton. Available at: https://pure.roehampton.ac.uk/portal/en/studentTheses/clinical-applications-of-the-polyvagal-theory-and-attachment-theory

Hastings, P. D., Nuselovici, J. N., Utendale, W. T., Coutya, J., McShane, K. E., & Sullivan, C. (2008). Applying the Polyvagal Theory to Children's Emotion Regulation: Social Context, Socialization, and Adjustment. *Biological Psychology*, 79(3), 299–306. https://doi.org/10.1016/j.biopsycho.2008.07.005

Heinonen, P., & Tainio, L. (2022). Intercorporeal Construction of We-Ness in Classroom Interaction. *Human Studies*. https://doi.org/10.1007/s10746-022-09659-x

Hillis, S., Ntwali N'konzi, J., Msemburi, W., Culver, L., Villaveces, A., Flaxman, S., & Unwin, H. J. T. (2022) Orphanhood and Caregiver Loss Among Children Based on New Global Excess COVID-19 Death Estimates. *JAMA Pediatrics* 2022 Nov; 176(11): 1145–1148 (Online) 10.1001/jamapediatrics.2022.3157

Hochleutner, K. (2018). Stuck in Somatic Countertransference: A Heuristic Study. *Creative Arts Therapies Theses*. 111. https://digitalcommons.colum.edu/theses_dmt/111

Huberman, A. (2022). *Using Play to Rewire & Improve Your Brain*. https://www.youtube.com/watch%3Fv%3DBwyZIWeBpRw&ved=2ahUKEwi3teXYop-FAxV2UUEAHcLoDfQQtwJ6BAgqEAI&usg=AOvVaw1b3LwA0BlDYCj4tTZUVLdS

Institute for Fiscal Studies. (2023). https://ifs.org.uk/sites/default/files/2023-07

Jennings, S. (1993). *Play Therapy with Children: A Practitioner's Guide*. Oxford: Wiley–Blackwell to Play Therapy.

Kestly, T. A. (2014). *The Interpersonal Neurobiology of Play: Brain-Building Interventions for Emotional Well-Being*. New York: W. W. Norton & Company, Inc.

Kolacz, J., daSilva, E. B., Lewis, G. F., Bertenthal, B. I., & Porges, S. W. (2021). Associations between Acoustic Features of Maternal Speech and infants' Emotion Regulation Following a Social Stressor. *Infancy*. https://doi.org/10.1111/infa.12440

Landreth, G. L. 2002. Play Therapy: The Art of the Relationship. 2nd ed. New York: Brunner-Routledge

LaPierre, A. (2015). Relational Body Psychotherapy (Or Relational Somatic Psychology. *International Body Psychotherapy Journal. The Art and Science of Somatic Praxis*, 14, 2.

LENA Foundation. (2022). https://www.lena.org/articles/babies-are-saying-less-since-the-pandemic-why-thats-concerning

Levine, P. A., & Kline, M. (2006). *Trauma through a Child's Eyes: Awakening the Ordinary Miracle of Healing*. California: Atlantic Books.

Lowry, C., Leonard-Kane, R., Gibbs, B., Muller, L. M., Peacock, A., & Jani, A. (2022). Teachers: the Forgotten Health Workforce. *Journal of the Royal Society of Medicine*, 115(4), 133–137. https://doi.org/10.1177/01410768221085692

Lucassen, N., Tharner, A., van IJzendoorn, M. H., Bakermans-Kranenburg, M. J., Volling, B. L., Hofman, A., & Tiemeier, H. (2010). *Paternal Sensitivity and History of Depression/Anxiety Predict Infant-Father Attachment Security* (Unpublished manuscript). The Netherlands: Leiden University.

Malchiodi, C. A. (2008). *Creative Interventions With Traumatized Children*. London: Guildford Press.

Maroda, K. J. (2004). *The Power of Countertransference: Innovations in Analytic Technique*. London: Analytic Press.

Maté, G., & Maté, D. (2022). *The myth of normal: trauma, illness & healing in a toxic culture*. New York, Avery, an imprint of Penguin Random House.

Mesman, J., et al. (2009). The Many Faces of the Still-Face Paradigm: A Review and Meta-Analysis. *Developmental Review*.

Murphy, F., et al. (2022) Childhood Trauma, the HPA Axis and Psychiatric Illnesses: A Targeted Literature Synthesis, Front. Psychiatry, 06 May 2022 Sec. Child and Adolescent Psychiatry Volume 13 - 2022 | https://doi.org/10.3389/fpsyt.2022.748372

Music, G., (2022). Resparking from Flatness: New Thoughts on Shut-Down States after Trauma and Neglect. *Journal of Child Psychotherapy*.

National Scientific Council on the Developing Child (2010). *Early Experiences Can Alter Gene Expression and Affect Long-Term Development:* Working Paper No. 10. http://www.developingchild.net

Newlove-Delgado, T., Marcheselli, F., Williams, T., Mandalia, D., Davis, J., McManus, S., Savic, M., Treloar, W., & Ford, T. (2022). *Mental Health of Children and Young People in England, 2022*. Leeds: NHS Digital.

Niedźwiecka, A. Eye Contact Effect: The Role of Vagal Regulation and Reactivity, and Self-Regulation of Attention. *Current Psychology* (2021). https://doi.org/10.1007/s12144-021-01682-y

Ofcom. (2020). Technology Tracker 2020. https://www.ofcom.org.uk/__data/assets/pdf_file/0037/194878/technology-tracker-2020-uk-data-tables.pdf

O'Neill, K. (2023). Symbolic Repair: A Model for Reparation in Non-Directive Play Therapy. Doctorate Thesis, Metanoia Institute.

Paley, B., & Hajal, N. J. (2022). Conceptualizing Emotion Regulation and Coregulation as Family-Level Phenomena. *Clinical Child and Family Psychology Review*, 25(1), 19–43. https://doi.org/10.1007/s10567-022-00378-4

Palmieri, A., Palvarini, V., Mangini, E., & Schimmenti, A. (2018). Transfert e Controtransfert Somatico: Rassegna critica e Integrazione Con La Prospettiva Neuroscientifica [Somatic Transference and Countertransference: A Critical Review and an Integration with the Neuroscientific Perspective]. *Rivista Di Psichiatria*, 53(6), 281–289.

Panksepp, J. (1998). *Affective Neuroscience: The Foundations of Human and Animal Emotions*. New York: Oxford University Press.

Panksepp, J. (2003). At the Interface of the Affective, Behavioural, and Cognitive Neurosciences: Decoding the Emotional Feelings of the Brain. *Brain and Cognition*, 52, 4–14.

Panksepp, J. (2007). Can PLAY Diminish ADHD and Facilitate the Construction of the Social Brain? *Journal of the Canadian Academy of Child and Adolescent Psychiatry*, 10, 57–66.

Perry, B. D. (1999). *"Memories of Fear: How the Brain Stores and Retrieves Physiologic States, Feelings, Behaviors and Thoughts from Traumatic Events"*. In J. M. Goodwin & R. Attias (Eds.), *Splintered Reflections: Images of the Body in Trauma* (pp. 26–47). Basic Books.

Perry, B. D. (2006). "Applying Principles of Neurodevelopment to Clinical Work With Maltreated and Traumatized Children: The Neurosequential Model of Therapeutics". In N. B. Webb (Ed.), *Working With Traumatized Youth in Child Welfare* (pp. 27–52). New York: The Guilford Press.

Porges, S. (2022). 'Our nervous system is always trying to figure out a way for us to survive, to be safe'. Interviewed by Kseib, K. *The British Psychological Society.* Accessed 23 November 2022. Available at: https://www.bps.org.uk/psychologist/our-nervous-system-always-trying-figure-out-way-us-survive-be-safe

Porges, S. W. (2003). Social Engagement and Attachment: a Phylogenetic Perspective. *Annals of the New York Academy of Sciences*, *1008*, 31–47. https://doi.org/10.1196/annals.1301.004

Porges, S. W. (2004). Neuroception: A Subconscious System for Detecting Threats and Safety. *Zero Three*, 24, 19–24.

Porges, S. W. (2007). The Polyvagal Perspective. *Biological Psychology*, 74(2), 116–143. https://doi.org/10.1016/j.biopsycho.2006.06.009

Porges, S. W. (2009). The Polyvagal Theory: New Insights into Adaptive Reactions of the Autonomic Nervous System. *Cleveland Clinic Journal of Medicine*, 76, S86–S90. https://doi.org/10.3949/ccjm.76.s2.17

Porges, S. W. (2011). *The Polyvagal Theory: Neurophysiological Foundations of Emotions, Attachment, Communication, Self-Regulation.* New York: W.W. Norton & Company.

Porges, S. W. (2015). Making the World Safe for our Children: Down-regulating Defence and Up-regulating Social Engagement to 'Optimise' the Human Experience. *Children Australia*, 40(2), 114–123. https://doi.org/10.1017/cha.2015.12

Porges, S. W. (2017). *The Pocket Guide to the Polyvagal Theory: The Transformative Power of Feeling Safe.* New York: W. W. Norton & Company.

Porges, S. W. (2017). *The Pocket Guide to the Polyvagal Theory: The Transformative Power of Feeling Safe.* London: W. W. Norton & Company.

Porges, S. W. (2021). Polyvagal Theory: A Biobehavioral Journey to Sociality. *Comprehensive Psychoneuroendocrinology*, 7, August 2021, 100069. https://doi.org/10.1016/j.cpnec.2021.100069

Porges S. W. (2022). Polyvagal Theory: A Science of Safety. *Frontiers in Integrative Neuroscience*, 16, 871227. https://doi.org/10.3389/fnint.2022.871227

Porges, S. W. (2023). The Vagal Paradox: A Polyvagal Solution. *Comprehensive Psychoneuroendocrinology*, 9(16), 100200.

Porges, S. W., & Dana, D. (2018). *Clinical Applications of the Polyvagal Theory – The Emergence of Polyvagal-Informed Therapies.* 1st ed. London: W. W. Norton & Company.

Porges, S. W., & Furman, S. A. (2011). The Early Development of the Autonomic Nervous System Provides a Neural Platform for Social Behavior: A Polyvagal Perspective. *Infant and Child Development*, 20(1), 106–118. https://doi.org/10.1002/icd.688

Porges, S. W., & Raskin, D. C. (1969). Respiratory and Heart Rate Components of Attention. *Journal of Experimental Psychology*, 81(3), 497–503. https://doi.org/10.1037/h0027921

Price, C. J., & Hooven, C. (2018). Interoceptive Awareness Skills for Emotion Regulation: Theory and Approach of Mindful Awareness in Body-Oriented Therapy (MABT). *Frontiers in Psychology*, 9, 798. https://doi.org/10.3389/fpsyg.2018.00798

Priddis, L., & Howieson, N. D. (2010). Transference and Attachment in Therapy and in Life. *Attachment: New Directions in Psychotherapy and Relational Psychoanalysis*, 4, 85–89.

Rand, M. L. (2003). Somatic Countertransference. (Somatic Resonance). Annals of the American Psychotherapy Association, 6(1), 48. https://link.gale.com/apps/doc/A99514105/AONE?u=googlescholar&sid=bookmark-AONE&xid=4aba5993

Rasic, D. (2010). Countertransference in Child and Adolescent Psychiatry: A Forgotten Concept? *Journal of the Canadian Academy of Child and Adolescent Psychiatry = Journal De l'Academie Canadienne De Psychiatrie De l'enfant Et De l'adolescent*, 19(4), 249–254.

Rosanbalm, K. D., & Murray, D. W. (2017). Promoting Self-Regulation in Early Childhood: A Practice Brief. OPRE Brief #2017-79. Washington, DC: Office of Planning, Research, and Evaluation, Administration for Children and Families, US. Department of Health and Human Services.

Russ, S. A. (2004). *Play in Child Development and Psychotherapy. Toward Empirically Supported Practice.* New Jersey: Lawrence Erlbaum Associates, Publishers.

Ryan, R. (2007). Motivation and Emotion: A New look and Approach for Two Re-Emerging Fields. *Motivation and Emotion*, 31, 1–3.

Sato, K., Fukai, T., Fujisawa, K. K., & Nakamuro, M.. Association between the COVID-19 Pandemic and Early Childhood Development. *JAMA Pediatrics*. Published online July 10, 2023. https://doi.org/10.1001/jamapediatrics.2023.2096

Save Our Children. (2020). https://www.savethechildren.org/content/dam/usa/reports/ed-cp/save-our-education

Schore, A. N. (1994). *Affect Regulation and the Origin of the Self: The Neurobiology of Emotional Development*. Hove: Lawrence Erlbaum Associates.

Schore, A. N. (2000). Attachment and the Regulation of the Right Brain. *Attachment & Human Development*, 2(1), 23–47. https://doi.org/10.1080/146167300361309

Schore, A. N. (2001). *Effects of a Secure Attachment Relationship on Right Brain Development, Affect Regulation, and Infant Mental Health. Infant Mental Health Journal*, 22(1–2), 7–66. https://doi.org/10.1002/1097-0355(200101/04)22:1<7::AID-IMHJ2>3.0.CO;2-N

Schore, A. N. (2005). A Neuropsychoanalytic Viewpoint: Commentary on Paper by Steven H. Knoblauch, *Psychoanalytic Dialogues*. https://doi.org/10.2513/s10481885pd1506_3

Schore, A. N. (2009). "Right-Brain Affect Regulation: An Essential Mechanism of Development, Trauma, Dissociation, and Psychotherapy". In D. Fosha, D. J. Siegel, & M. F. Solomon (Eds.), *The Healing Power of Emotion: Affective Neuroscience, Development & Clinical Practice* (pp. 112–144). New York: W. W. Norton & Company.

Schore, J., & Schore, A. (2007). Modern Attachment Theory: The Central Role of Affect Regulation in Development and Treatment. *Clinical Social Work Journal*, 36, 9–20. https://doi.org/10.1007/s10615-007-0111-7

Schore, J. R., & Schore, A. N. (2008). Modern Attachment Theory: The Central Role of Affect Regulation in Development and Treatment. *Clinical Social Work Journal*, 36, 9–20.

Schwartz, A. (2018) Connection and Co-Regulation in Psychotherapy, www.drarielleschwartz.com. Accessed 6th April 2023. Available at: https://drarielleschwartz.com/connection-co-regulation-psychotherapy-dr-arielle-schwartz/#.ZBwgk3bP25c

Sege, R., Bethell, C., Linkenbach, J., Jones, J., Klika, B., & Pecora, P. J. (2017). *Balancing Adverse Childhood Experiences with HOPE: New Insights into the Role of Positive Experience on Child and Family Development*. Boston: The Medical Foundation.

Shatz, C. J. (1992). The Developing Brain. *Scientific American*, *267*(3), 60–67.

Siegel, D., & Sroufe, L. A. (2011). The Verdict Is in: The Case for Attachment Theory. Accessed 7th October 2023. Available at: https://drdansiegel.com/wp-content/uploads/2020/09/1271-the-verdict-is-in-1.pdf

Siegel, D. J. (1999). *The Developing Mind: Toward a Neurobiology of Interpersonal Experience*. New York: Guilford Press.

Siegel, D. J., & Payne Bryson, T. (2011). *The Whole-Brain Child: 12 Revolutionary Strategies to Nurture Your Child's Developing Mind*. Bantam Books.

Slade, A. (2005). Parental Reflective Functioning: an Introduction. *Attachment & Human Development*, 7(3), 269–281. https://doi.org/10.1080/14616730500245906

Sleater, A., & Scheinerb, (2019). The Impact of the Therapist's "Use of Self". *The European Journal of Counselling Psychology*.

Soma, C. S., Baucom, B. R. W., Xiao, B., Butner, J. E., Hilpert, P., Narayanan, S., Atkins, D. C., & Imel, Z. E. (2020). Coregulation of Therapist and Client Emotion During Psychotherapy. *Psychotherapy Research*, 30(5), 591–603. https://doi.org/10.1080/10503307.2019.1661541

Sroufe, A. (1996). *Emotional Development: The Organization of Emotional Life in the Early Years*. New York: Cambridge University Press.

Stevens, V. (2014). To Think Without Thinking: The Implications of Combinatory Play and the Creative Process for Neuroaesthetics. *American Journal of Play*, Fall *2014*, 99–119.

Stone, M. (2006). The analyst's Body as Tuning Fork: Embodied Resonance in Countertransference. *The Journal of Analytical Psychology*, 51(1), 109–124. https://doi.org/10.1111/j.1465-5922.2006.575_1.x

Sunderland, M. (2000). *Using Story Telling as a Therapeutic Tool With Children*. London: Speechmark Publishing Ltd.

Sutanti, N. (2020). Understanding Congruence in Person-Centred Counselling Practice: A Trainee Counsellor's Perspective, *Journal of Professionals in Guidance and Counseling*, 1(2), 2020, 47–55. https://doi.org/10.21831/progcouns.v1i2.34615

Tierney, A. L., & Nelson, C. A. 3rd (2009). Brain Development and the Role of Experience in the Early Years. *Zero to Three*, 30(2), 9–13.

Tronick, E., & Beeghly, M. (2011). Infants' Meaning-Making and the Development of Mental Health Problems. *The American Psychologist*, 66(2), 107–119. https://doi.org/10.1037/a0021631

Tsarkova, A. (2015). *Exploring clinicians' experience of countertransference in play therapy*. Masters Thesis, Smith College, Northampton, MA. https://scholarworks.smith.edu/theses/669

Tucci, J., Weller, A., & Mitchell, J. (2018). "Realizing "deep" Safety for Children Who Have Experienced Abuse: Application of Polyvagal Theory in Therapeutic Work with Traumatized Children and Young People". In S. W. Porges & D. Dana (Eds.), *Clinical Applications of the Polyvagal Theory: The Emergence of Polyvagal-Informed Therapies* (pp. 89–105). London: W. W. Norton & Company.

UNESCO. (2021). *Education: From disruption to recovery: Covid-19 Impact on Education*. https://en.unesco.org/covid19/educationresponse

van der Kolk, B. A. (2009). Entwicklungstrauma-störung: Auf dem weg zu einer sinnvollen diagnostik für chronisch traumatisierte kinder [Developmental Trauma Disorder: Towards a Rational Diagnosis for Chronically Traumatized Children]. *Praxis der Kinderpsychologie und Kinderpsychiatrie*, 58(8), 572–586. https://doi.org/10.13109/prkk.2009.58.8.572

Wagner, D. (2015). Polyvagal Theory and Peek-a-Boo: How the Therapeutic Pas De Deux Heals Attachment Trauma. *Body, Movement and Dance in Psychotherapy*, 10(4), 256–265. https://doi.org/10.1080/17432979.2015.1069762

Wheeler, N., & Dillman Taylor, D. (2016). Integrating Interpersonal Neurobiology With Play Therapy. *International Journal of Play Therapy*, 25, 24–34.

Whitehead, C. C. (2006). Psychoanalysis: A Paradigm for the 21st Century. *Journal of the Academy of Psychoanalysis and Dynamic Psychiatry*, 34, 603–627.

Winnicott, D. W. (1953). Transitional Objects and Transitional Phenomena; a Study of the First Not-Me Possession. *The International Journal of Psychoanalysis*, 34, 89–97.

Winnicott, D. W. (1966). Psycho-somatic Illness in Its Positive and Negative Aspects. *The International Journal of Psychoanalysis*, 47(4), 510–516.

Wise, J. (2022). Covid-19: Babies born during the pandemic show slight development delays. *British Medical Journal*, 376:o29. https://doi.org/10.1136/bmj.o29

World Health Organization (2020). *Naming the coronavirus disease (COVID-19) and the virus that causes it* https://www.who.int/emergencies/diseases/novel-coronavirus-2019/technical-guidance/naming-the-coronavirus-disease-(covid-2019)-and-the-virus-that-causes-it

World Health Organization (2023). *COVID-19 weekly epidemiological update*. Edition 135 published 22 March 2023. https://www.who.int/publications

Index